BUT I HARDLY EVER SNEEZE

What You Don't Know Could Kill You

Brain Fog

Fatigue

Back Pain

Asthma

Restless Legs

Obesity

Unexplained Sadness, Anger, and Depression

Tollie Moore DeGraw

outskirts press

But I Hardly Ever Sneeze
What You Don't Know Could Kill You
All Rights Reserved.
Copyright © 2019 Tollie Moore DeGraw
v1.0

The opinions expressed in this manuscript are solely the opinions of the author and do not represent the opinions or thoughts of the publisher. The author has represented and warranted full ownership and/or legal right to publish all the materials in this book.

This book may not be reproduced, transmitted, or stored in whole or in part by any means, including graphic, electronic, or mechanical without the express written consent of the publisher except in the case of brief quotations embodied in critical articles and reviews.

Outskirts Press, Inc.
http://www.outskirtspress.com

ISBN: 978-1-9772-1283-2

Cover Photo © 2019 www.gettyimages.com. All rights reserved - used with permission.

Outskirts Press and the "OP" logo are trademarks belonging to Outskirts Press, Inc.

PRINTED IN THE UNITED STATES OF AMERICA

*To Dr. Marek Maria Pienkowski, brilliant physician
who has saved my life in more ways than he will ever know*

Preface

ALLERGY-RELATED ILLNESSES PREDATE my earliest childhood memories, and the allergic condition has come to define my life. I was naïve and clueless for a very long time as mysterious symptoms would come and go, seemingly of their own free will. My life was a puzzle of massive proportions. After decades of searching for missing pieces, this giant life-sized jigsaw puzzle has finally been solved. I faced naysayers, doubters, skeptics and deniers, but I was never deterred. I always had faith that the answers would come. I just didn't know it would take me 40 years to find them.

As I finally became healthy enough to write this book, the words flowed freely and it practically wrote itself. I am eager and determined to share with the world all my personal details as the pieces finally came together to frame my newfound healthy life.

Depression, backache, restless legs, digestive issues, brain fog, lethargy and chronic bronchitis are just a few of the myriad of symptoms which plagued me off and on for many years and have now thankfully diminished into distant memories.

Throughout my early journey I was misled, misinformed, misread, misunderstood and dismissed, but not intentionally. That all changed when I met Dr. Pienkowski. He was my turning point. He introduced me to the complexities of allergy and he healed me.

This book is not meant to be just another self-help instructional manual. It is an emotional and riveting story about a young woman whose allergies altered her life by providing unwelcome and often painful twists and turns for years and years. These mysterious health issues have provided extraordinary knowledge, insight, and a perspective that the general public has yet to realize. My intention is to encourage healing and enhance awareness by offering examples and solutions which have worked so well for me throughout the years.

I am uniquely qualified to tell my story. Thousands of hours of research, journaling, and recording consistent cause-and-effect results simply cannot be denied.

Only I know what I could have been had I not come face-to-face with all these various allergic monsters on an almost daily basis. One thing, however, is clearly true. I never could have mustered the strength and courage to fight a single battle without the love and support of a devoted and faithful husband. He is my rock.

As I write this book, I am reminded of a poem I memorized in some English class long ago. The words of Emily Dickinson ring true to me still, as I try to define my purpose.

She wrote,

> "If I can stop one heart from breaking,
> I shall not live in vain;
> If I can ease one life the aching,
> Or cool one pain,
> Or help one fainting robin
> Unto his nest again,
> I shall not live in vain."[1]

---

1   Dickenson, Emily, The Complete Poems of Emily Dickenson. Boston: Little, Brown, 1924. Bartleby.com. July 20, 2018. www.bartleby.com/113/.

Acknowledgements

MY LIFELONG DETERMINATION to someday publish the details of my all-too-often misunderstood allergic episodes could never have come to fruition without the love, encouragement and support of so many people with whom I have shared encounters along the way. Many faces and common experiences have faded through the years, yet their stories remain uplifting and I offer my heartfelt appreciation to all who have touched my life. For certain, God's Hand has always led the way, and for that I am eternally grateful.

To Michael, whose patience and abiding love secured our future, you are truly my soul and inspiration. Thank you for being you.

To Dr. Linda Best, professor and editor extraordinaire, who has been teaching and advising for as long as I have been searching for answers, thank you for the education you have provided me in these few short months. Your wise counsel and editing expertise are unparalleled in their value.

To our daughter, Jennifer, whose generous nature supports me in every facet of my life, I thank you for being my creative go-to-girl for all things, literary and otherwise. You are my second heartbeat, and without your devotion to my well-being, our story could never have made it to the printed page.

To our loving grandson, Joshua, who has learned more about computers in his thirteen years than I can hope to learn in my lifetime, thank you for sharing your technical skills, especially in creating the Word Board. I could not have designed it without your enthusiastic help.

To all my extended family and adopted friends, thank you for putting up with my unpredictable and quirky ways throughout the years. To borrow a phrase from grandson Parker, "You are DeGrawsome."

And finally, to my parents, who continue to guide, inspire, and encourage me from up in Heaven, I forgive you for naming me "Clyde," because "It was stylish back in the day to give boys' names to our daughters." Surely you must have been allergified! Wish you were here to laugh together and celebrate our success.

Prologue

ALLERGIES ARE TRICKY little things. They can make you crazy. Or at least they make you feel as if you are. Tiny little symptom-causing allergens float around in the air you breathe and hide in the food you eat. They sneak up on you and invade your space. They make your back hurt. They creep into your brain and make you angry. They make you cry on your happiest days. They make you fat. They make you panic, and they phobatize you. They make your chest produce creepy little wheezy sounds. They choke you and make you cough. They sniffle you up and cause loud scary vibrating noises when you sleep. They monopolize you and make you sad. They give you geographic tongue and they erase your libido. They are uninvited and unexpected guests. They wreak havoc and create mayhem. They put you to sleep when you want to be awake. They keep you awake when you need to be asleep. They tingle your hands and numb your fingertips. They are unexplainable and unpredictable. They cause food cravings. They jump out and attack your insides when you eat them. They mimic other things.

They change your handwriting and they fog up your brain. They flush you out and bind you up. They are illusive and they make your hair fall out. They blow up your abdomen like a balloon. They crack your heels and make you itchy. They swell up your lips and stop up your ears. They try to smell good, and they make you puffy. They like soft places and they like to hide. They splotch up your skin. They heat up your cheeks and your earlobes. They defy logic and put you in a trance. They make your legs get all twitchy. They stop up your nose and they water your eyes. They crackle your ears and they make your throat itch. They soak up your energy and dull your sense of taste and smell. They make your muscles and your joints ache. They blur your vision and cross your eyes. They upset your stomach and make you moody. They raise bumps on your skin, they steal your time, and they mess with your memory. They have to be outsmarted and they have to be avoided. But before you can avoid them, you have to identify them. They are powerful. They can kill you...

And every little once in a while, they make you sneeze.

Introduction

I WILL ALWAYS remember the summer of my sixty-third year. That's when I got my brain back.

Unsolved mysteries, unanswered questions, illogical responses, unpredictable reactions, unexplainable behaviors, seemingly undiagnosable medical conditions and obesity have defined my life for as long as I can remember.

These unwelcome tyrants have been constantly lurking in my shadows for well over 40 years. Like Sherlock Holmes, Miss Marple and Nancy Drew, I have been working the puzzle and solving the mysteries, piece by piece and clue by clue. Today I truly understand the link between allergy, emotions, behavior, and pain. I have chased away the uninvited monsters and most of my mysteries are solved. Sixty pounds lighter than I was just a few short years ago, I am completely de-sensitized and obesity no longer rules my body or my mind.

I am not a doctor, I am not a scientist, and I am not associated with any products or services. I cannot even say that what has worked for me will also work for you. That is for you alone to decide. What I am is an expert on myself. I have a story to tell and an overwhelming desire to help others by sharing the knowledge I have gained along the way. The statistics and percentages to which I refer are timely and accurate as well as I can determine. They are meant to be used only as a general reference to illustrate various scenarios and to help the reader put things in perspective. This testimonial is a personal account of my lifelong struggle as I have emerged from the depths of severe allergic disease into a happy, healthy symptom-free life.

As I began the process of healing, my initial goals had nothing to do with writing a book. I just wanted to get well. The details of my journey are taken from my personal experiences and based only on my own notes, journals, observations and research accumulated since I first met my allergist, Dr. Marek Pienkowski. It comes from my heart in hopes that I can help raise public awareness as to what it really means to have an allergic constitution. This book is my light at the end of a very long tunnel.

In the beginning stages, treating the obvious symptoms relating to food allergy and allergic rhinitis was rooted in basic medical science. I started feeling better right away. The vague physical and emotional problems which lay beneath the surface were another matter entirely. It didn't take me 40 years to solve my mysteries because I wasn't smart enough. Quite the contrary. My IQ of 147 wasn't even enough to see through all the obstacles in my path. I graduated near the top of my class from one of the best high schools in America in 1965. I studied French and journalism at the University of North Carolina at Greensboro and pictured myself as a glamorous foreign correspondent. It was not to be.

As I was growing up, medical science was just beginning to consider new approaches to old problems. Many professionals in the medical community were unprepared to recognize the allergy connection as it related to my ongoing complaints. Not that they didn't believe me, but rather that this complex concept was as yet unrecognized and therefore not part of the medical school curriculum. My personal search for answers has been extensive and extremely rewarding. Many of my findings will astound you.

Often through the years I have been difficult to live with. It was never on purpose. My tears were seldom over any real issues and my weight gain was never the result of hiding Oreos under the bed. I have suffered with bouts of chronic bronchitis, year-round allergies, asthma and flu-like symptoms for most of my adult life. I have had painful back problems, mood-swings and quickly-changing episodes of anger and joy, sadness and euphoria, combined with complicated aches and pains which mimic a myriad of other diseases.

The only accurate diagnosis I have ever received is that my various symptoms and illnesses are all allergy-related. As I uncover and identify the clues which have helped me along the way, I hope you discover an equally successful path of your own, one not previously taken, and maybe one not even remotely considered. Anything is possible, but one thing is certain. You can't change something you don't recognize and acknowledge. My "Aha!" moments have been significant and enduring. Many say that allergy has no cure, and technically speaking perhaps they are right. I beg to differ.

Whether your life is a huge jagged-edged uncompleted puzzle or whether you are simply looking for one small missing piece, perhaps you will find it here as you read your way through these pages which represent my struggle in search of "normalcy." I have found my answers and you can find yours. "Aha!" moments are almost always followed by success. I wish you Godspeed.

Table of Contents

The quandaries, hurdles and puzzles of my life

Allergic Disease
WHAT IS ALLERGY?
#youthinkyouknowbutyouprobablyreallydon't

Allergies were first identified around 400 B.C. by the Greek philosopher and physician Hippocrates. He observed that some people, but not all, were allergic to cheese. About 350 years later the Roman philosopher Lucretius wrote that "What is food to one person may be bitter poison to others." The specific word "allergy" was introduced in 1906 by an Australian pediatrician, Clemens Von Perquet to describe undesired reactions to food and other substances.

Allergy is a synonym for hypersensitivity, and it is subject to various interpretations. An abnormal reaction of the immune system, it occurs as a response to otherwise harmless substances. In general terms, it refers to a strong aversion to something. Allergy can be caused by almost any substance in the universe. That which causes the response is an allergen, and the substance itself is a trigger. When reactions occur in sequence it is called "piling on."

Fifty million Americans are affected by some form of allergic disorder. Many more are not even aware that they fall into this category. Allergy is the sixth leading cause of chronic disease in the United States. Help is available if you know where to find it.

Although you don't inherit an allergy to a specific substance, you can inherit the tendency to be allergic. If both your parents are allergic, the chances are that you are too. If you and your spouse are both allergic, odds are that your children will be as well. People are either allergic or they are not. It is not a matter of opinion. If you toss a handful of pollen into a person's face, he or she will either cough and sneeze or calmly wipe away the pollen. If you are a sneezer, the only way to identify your triggers is to be professionally tested by a certified allergist. I strongly advise you to do so.

My children came up with a term of their own when they were teenagers in the 1980's. One time when I was having a really difficult and frustrating allergic day, Jennifer said to Andy, "Don't bother Mom. She's allergified." It was a perfect description and has been applied to my condition more times than I can count throughout the following years. It is an excellent word, and to those of you who yourselves have ever been allergified, you know exactly what I am talking about. Thankfully, I seldom hear the word pertaining to myself anymore and that too is a most excellent thing.

So we have defined allergy in medical terms and we have defined allergy in layman's terms. Now it is time to define allergy in my terms:

MONSTERS!!!

Physicians and scientists make a clear distinction between a true allergic response and sensitivity. Scientifically, the first allergic exposure induces the production of protective substances called Immunoglobulin E (IgE) antibodies. They travel to mast cells which then release chemicals such as histamines to fight the invading allergens. Subsequent exposures trigger the release of an array of chemicals (mediators of sensitivity) which then act on other cells, producing symptoms. When you have an allergy, the immune system is involved. Sensitivity is largely triggered in the digestive system or other parts of the body. If you have an allergic constitution, you are susceptible to an infinite number of reactions. Examples of common allergens are pollen, food, mold, latex, insect stings, dust mites, and pet dander. The list of possible allergens is endless.

The following seven categories illustrate examples of various sources of allergens and how we are exposed to them.

1. Contactants are any allergens which cause a reaction by coming into contact with skin or mucous membranes. Examples are cosmetics, lipstick, chap stick, fabrics, plant oils, soap, lotions, chemicals such as formaldehyde, latex, and metals such as the nickel found in jewelry.

2. Ingestants include such items as food, drugs, spices, beverages, colorings, additives, chewing gum, paints (especially on children's toys, not only lead-based), smoke, and anything else which passes through the lips.

3. Injectants are vaccines, serum, drugs by injection, insect bites and stings, animal bites, and anything else which pierces the skin.

4. Inhalents are airborne particles we breathe, such as pollen, dust, powder, hair spray, molds, dander from people or animals, feathers, chemical fumes from substances such as gasoline, perfume, paint, mothballs, candles, air fresheners, aerosol sunscreens, and smoke.

5. Molds and fungi can cause reactions by inhalation, ingestion, or contact. Examples are penicillin, yeast, mildew and mushrooms.

6. Physical conditions such as heat, cold, dampness, sunlight, drafts, and mechanical irritation such as scratches, irritation, and wounds can also cause allergic reactions.

7. Allergy can also be caused by infectious agents, such as germs and bacteria used in tuberculin and other medical diagnostic testing.

Allergic reactions can be lessened and even corrected by desensitization (immunizations) and omitted by avoidance but there is no perfect cure. When you acquire tolerance for one substance, you may then acquire sensitivity to another. Some childhood allergies can be outgrown, but adult onset allergies can appear at any time. If left unattended, they can become a contributing factor to lots of other health issues, especially in later life when for various reasons allergy medications are no longer possible. Immunization, however, is an option at any age.

When allergies do occur, reactions are controlled by the central nervous system, which governs such things as the tear ducts, salivary glands, respiratory organs, digestive system, and the heart. Swelling can occur anywhere in the body, including the brain. When allergens attack the emotional centers of the brain, it seems only logical to me that the result could be an abundance of unexplained feelings and behaviors. These seemingly irrational and mysterious reactions can easily interfere with interpersonal relationships. The accompanying frustrations can then snowball into issues resulting in such things as depression, low self-esteem and even guilt. Children as well as adults can be affected. The emotional turmoil is made even worse when those around them are uninformed, misinformed, and as a possible result, insensitive.

Recognizing the primary layer of allergy is easy. The signs and symptoms of congestion and pain are fairly obvious. Recognizing the multitude of secondary layers is another matter entirely. Even though each of our body parts is a separate unit, the symptoms affecting them overlap and do not occur separately. It is a symbiotic relationship. Only an allergist who is committed to treating the whole body rather than individual symptoms will be able to identify the profound significance of these secondary layers which lay buried beneath the sneezes.

Sadly in my opinion, some doctors are reluctant to refer their patients to an allergist. They prefer to treat the symptoms as they appear and re-appear. Too often it is easier to write a prescription than it is to search out the cause. If there are mysteries in your life, I urge you to get tested so you know for sure. This is true for children as well.

Throughout my story, I will be using the word "allergy" in a general sense. The ability to cause upheaval is very real, whether the reaction is the result of sensitivity or a true allergic response. I am not really sure that the medical definition even matters to the average person. My symptoms overlapped to the extent that for me it was impossible to differentiate between the two. Therefore, "allergy" will refer to any reaction to substances in the environment which create a negative modification in my physical being, my emotions, or my behavior.

Most allergy-related signs and symptoms are easily recognized and treatable. Many are not. Hopefully as you follow my journey and realize how complex some of the issues are, you will have your own "light bulb moment" which will shorten your search for success as you identify the allergy connection. Through the years it has become clear to me that many, many people do not really understand the complexities of allergy at all, and the skeptics are hard to convince. They may think that "Everyone has allergies. What is the big deal?" If this is your experience, it may become necessary for you to dig deep and recognize the patterns for yourself. I hope the tools I am providing will be helpful.

Going forward, I find myself on a mission of compassion, born of a giving spirit and a strong desire to educate and explain by relating what I have learned along the way. I believe in the old adage that to those whom much is given, much is expected. I have an intriguing story to tell. Some of it may be hard to accept, and you are not required to do so, but it is a true and accurate account of what allergy has meant to me. At any rate, my complicated story has a happy ending and I am convinced that sharing its components will contribute to the Greater Good.

FINDING DR. P.

#thereisananswerafterall

The path to my success began back in the 1980's. I was always sick, and nothing seemed to help. I was gaining weight, constantly tired and irritable, and my illness was taking its toll on the family. I was a mess and every little thing turned into an infection. On the advice of a concerned cousin, I made an appointment with an aller-gist, Dr. Marek Maria Pienkowski. A soft- spoken man of Polish de-scent, his credentials were impeccable and his reputation was stellar. As a respected diagnostician, he focused on health issues involving allergies and the immune system. He was involved in research and he was solving mysteries. Little did I realize it at the time, but my life was about to change. From the moment of our first introduction, I was finally on the path to recovery.

I was surprised to find out that my first visit was more of a consul-tation than a physical examination. Rather than immediately listening to my wheezing chest, peering into my stopped-up ears and drippy nose and telling me I was congested (which of course I already knew), he welcomed me into his spacious office, and directed me to a com-fortable chair across from him at his beautiful spacious desk which consisted of an uncluttered gleaming slab of smooth hard granite, ele-gantly non-allergenic. He wanted me to tell him about my symptoms, everything that was bothering me. Every detail was important, and I wasn't to leave anything out. Slowly, and a little hesitantly at first, I began describing the roller coaster ride that had become my life. I was an emotional and physical wreck. I didn't know where to turn. Tears began to spill down over my cheeks as I told him my story. He listened intently for over an hour, nodding his head and encouraging me to continue. After assuring me that he really heard me and did not think any of this was all in my head, he offered me a box of tissues. I cannot begin to describe the relief I felt as I sat there in his office that day. Someone finally understood what I was talking about.

He had a plan. He tested me for all kinds of allergies. He tested my thyroid, my blood, everything imaginable, and he ordered an ultra-sound examination of my heart. He was ruling out other condi-tions, one by one. Now I understand even more what he was doing. He was searching for clues.

A week or so later, when all the test results were in, I returned to the chair in his office. He was smiling. After a few pleasantries (designed, I am sure, to put me at ease), Dr. Pienkowski spoke the following magical words. They have sustained me throughout this long process and they are permanently etched in my heart. He said,

"Mrs. DeGraw, the only thing keeping you from running the marathon is allergy-related."

I was stunned. Again, tears began streaming down my face, only this time they were happy tears. Tears of relief. I did not have some dreaded disease. I wasn't destined for a mental hospital or to a life of chronic pain. I wasn't dying, and my life wasn't over. I had severe allergic disease and it could be treated. Again he passed me the tissue box, and we both smiled.

Without a doubt, we now know that his diagnosis was spot on. Despite my decades of turmoil, there has never been another explanation. There is still no cure for the allergic condition, but symptoms can be treated, lessened, and even eliminated. I am living proof that there are answers out there. You just have to find them. Everything Dr. Pienkowski prescribed and suggested has worked and is still working. Without his accurate diagnosis, I never would have been able to connect all of my unusual symptoms to allergy. The sneeze, a telltale sign of allergy to most people, was buried among my huge conglomeration of complaints, and I hardly ever noticed it at all.

I began my mission by taking a few edge pieces out of the puzzle box. Gradually the frame took shape and I set out to complete it, one ragged piece at a time. My determination was unfaltering. It came from somewhere deep within my soul. I felt like a small boat in a big ocean with no one else on board. Progress was episodic. I would make great strides then meet with an obstacle I couldn't define. The seas calmed when Dr. Pienkowski took the helm.

We set out immediately on a plan of education, avoidance, immunizations and proper medications. I went to the library and came home with a stack of books which reached from the floor all the way up to my chin. Determined to find all the answers and reclaim my healthy happy life, my journey began. I sat on the floor in the middle of the living room, with all these books spread out around me and I was mesmerized. Here and there I found familiar snippets and stories. Almost immediately I realized that little was actually known about the relationship between allergy, emotions, behavior and pain. It wasn't something physicians studied in medical school. Every situation was different and nothing could be proven consistently. It was too complicated. I was on my own. Little did I know that it would take decades for me to finally put it all together and become healthy enough to share my successful discoveries by writing this book.

From the beginning of my treatment phase, I was motivated to keep journals, memos, magazine articles and observations, even though sometimes the words were merely scribbled notes on torn pieces of paper. I wasn't thinking of a book. I was just trying to get well by peeling the proverbial onion, layer by layer. Since there was no internet, information was sketchy. Even in this information age, I find that still to be the case. Thankfully I didn't throw my scribbles away.

MY SYMPTOMS
#symptomsaresignsofsomethingstrangewhichotherssometimescannotsee

Medically speaking, symptoms can only be described by the person feeling them. If you have pain, chances are that no one knows about it unless you tell them. Signs are indicators of a problem as seen through the eyes of others. At times I have been frustrated when others sympathize with my rashes, coughing, and congestion but are unable to comprehend the internal turmoil which often accompanies these conditions. I attributed their reactions to a lack of empathy on their part. I was wrong. I did not understand the difference between signs and symptoms from another person's point of view. I expected others to understand and sympathize with what I barely understood myself.

If your back itches, no one will know unless they see you scratching. The unknown internal symptom only becomes a known sign when it is recognized externally. So many of us don't like to complain, but if we don't speak out, we are only delaying the healing process. The backscratcher has always been one of my favorite inventions. There is one in almost every room of our house, even pretty and unusual antiques. However, I must admit that Michael is the best backscratcher of all. He gets plenty of practice! Now that most of my itches have disappeared, my collection of backscratchers is mostly just decorative but I can't part with any of them, just in case. Recognizing and eliminating our illusive symptoms would be so much easier if there were tools for every one of them!

Obese people are often stereotyped as having no will power and no desire to exercise. The overweight signs are obvious, just by looking. In my case there were and still are many mysterious internal symptoms fighting against all my efforts to lose weight. Forces were working against me in ways that can still be difficult to understand. The signs and symptoms were at odds with each other and because of allergy, unknown to me at the time, I always felt as if I were fighting a losing battle. Casual observers could never understand, but I hope to encourage compassion and to help diminish these undeserved labels.

For the sake of speaking in laymen's terms I will use the words "signs" and "symptoms" interchangeably, even though there really is a difference.

There is no doubt that my allergic experiences have had a large impact on those closest to me. The fact that they are interspersed with relatively healthy periods and an exceptionally stable home life has made any consistently accurate self-diagnosis practically impossible. If any of the following symptoms are familiar to you, then you know that when a family member struggles with severe sporadic, unexplainable episodes, the process takes an emotional toll on the lives of those who love them.

Many of my symptoms have coincided with those associated with Chronic Fatigue Syndrome. It is said that more than half of the CFS patients studied suffer from allergies, yet testing is not always considered in the diagnosis. The same is true for Irritable Bowel Syndrome, Depression, and Fibromyalgia. I don't understand why the allergy factor is so often trivialized or even ignored in illnesses such as these. For us, this quest for knowledge has been exasperating, to say the least.

The good news is that when all is said and done, I am living proof that answers can be found.

The following symptoms have haunted me at various times throughout my life. There are probably even more which I have already forgotten. If any are familiar to you and you have discovered no cure and no logical explanation for their existence, follow along with me and maybe you too can recognize a possible solution not previously considered. With the exception of the few remaining symptoms mentioned afterward, these conditions are no longer a part of my life. These monsters followed me around in random order, creating mayhem, season after season, year after year, and decade after decade. They gradually disappeared along with my allergies, as my health continued to improve and I am eager to share the successful process with all of you.

For years I suffered with –

aphasia tingling anger
asthma cravings burping
shiners dizziness bloating earache
dandruff drowsiness confusion fatigue
headache candidiasis sinusitis
panic arthritis conjuctivitis SAD edema
itching rhinitis irritability brainfog RLS
hearturn puffiness bronchitis cravings
IBS backache depression wheezing
moodiness spasms
yawning lethargy UTI sunbumps
thrush rashes

The few remaining obstacles preventing a perfectly symptom-free life are minimal and easily manageable. They include occasional abdominal swelling, usually related to food allergy or chemical exposure, which causes the numbers on the scale to fluctuate abundantly; recognizable emotional reactions related to chemical sensitivity; candida albicans symptoms such as rash and food cravings, related to changes in diet; and sun allergy, controllable by limiting exposure.

If you are surprised that I am connecting all these symptoms to allergy, you are not alone. Everyone knows allergy means sneezing, itchy watery eyes, running noses, and congestion. Springtime miseries caused by pollen are followed by another sneezy season in the fall.

Television commercials bombard us constantly with every possible over-the-counter medication. Antihistamines, decongestants, cough syrups, ointments, nasal sprays and eye drops are guaranteed to totally eliminate our miserable allergy symptoms. That is, until they re-appear and we have to run out and buy more of the same products, along with tissues, aspirin and ibuprofen. It is a multi-billion dollar business, but it is not my business. I am not against these products. Medications were necessary as I began my treatment. It is just that there are answers beyond pill-popping. I believe it is time we dig down and find the cause of all this misery and quit putting Band-Aids on the problems. In my personal situation, I found that sometimes the same medicines which were supposed to be helping me were actually adding to my complex symptoms. I will explain later.

There is another concept involved in understanding the enormous influence that allergy has on the immune system and the body's overall healthy status. Referred to as the Allergic (or Atopic) March, it pertains to the progression of various allergic symptoms as they develop in sequence as we age. Apparently, the first decade of a person's life is significant because the incidence of allergic responses and diseases related to the immune system is higher during these years than at any other time in life. Sensitivity to environmental allergens is increasingly identified during the preschool years.

As the march continues, our bodies switch from one atopic

expression of allergy to another. As we approach puberty, hormones become a contributing factor. Interleukins (hormones of the immune system) appear, triggering the release of histamines and other inflammatory chemicals. It is much like a chain reaction, with one reaction leading to the next as the years go by. Extensive research on this subject has emerged in the last couple of decades and once I became familiar with the process of allergic progression, it became clear to me that my life mirrors this scientific theory in great detail. From infancy through my senior years, I have been marching in step. We need to find out how to halt the march. Scientists are trying, and I wish them Godspeed.

My Story
#wishingyouwellandhopingyouwillfindyouranswershere

As the soft first light of morning tiptoes gently over the foothills, it slowly spills into the valley and the morning chorus begins. Mocking birds lead the choir here in eastern Tennessee, and the glory of it all exhilarates me. There was a time when I would have missed the symphony. I would have been cowering inside, trying not to breathe the air. But not today. Spring arrives majestically in our small town. Pollen covers the cars and patios and lays down a floating yellow carpet over Melton Hill Lake. Dogwoods are in bloom as lime green leaf tips make their appearance among the fading white flowers of the Bradford Pears. Fluffy round puffs of pollen from the Sycamore trees are dancing through the air and Maple tree helicopters are twirling all around me.

The sounds of coughing, sneezing, sniffling and wheezing throughout the congregation competed with the words of the sermon on Sunday morning. As I listened to the familiar indications of the spring allergy season, an inner peace rose up around me as I celebrated my silence in the sanctuary. I too am allergic, yet here I sit today, writing this book in my garden, savoring the sweet perfume of the pink and purple hyacinths at my feet as the budding tendrils of honeysuckle wind their way around the tree behind my bench. Overcome by the joy of simply being here, bare toes wiggling among the violets and cool green grass, I can take it all in, breathing deeply, and I am not sick.

Life wasn't always this way.

The one true thread that weaves itself constantly in and out of my story is one that might surprise you. You see, more than anything else, this book is a love story.

I married the love of my life 49 years ago in 1968. Together we have been on a roller coaster of up-days and down-days, attacking monsters of unknown origins and searching for explanations when there were none. Our love has never faltered and Michael always makes me smile. His devotion is unquestionable and our wedding vows have remained a sacred commitment through all these years. Little did we know that the phrase "in sickness and in health" would become an oxymoron, as these two conditions have followed us around simultaneously throughout all the days of our lives. Michael has been my consistent inspiration and my constant love. He has always been my source of energy and I still find it difficult to comprehend when he says he gets his energy from me.

A lucrative lifelong career may not have been God's plan for me, but loving and supportive friends and family have filled my heart with gold. Today we have reached the end of the roller coaster track and we are smiling on level ground. I look forward to what the future brings as our story continues to unfold.

Allergies have been part of my life since birth, when as a baby I came close to death from a severe reaction to penicillin. Gradually increasing in its power over my mind and body, seasonal allergy became severe allergic disease, complicated by food allergy and chemical sensitivity. They turned my life upside down and created in me a person whose thoughts, emotions, and behaviors were unpredictable and often unavoidable. I didn't recognize myself. In an instant I could change from my usual cheerful disposition to being upset about something, and feeling inside like I was someone I didn't even know, and really didn't even like very much.

By the time I reached my mid-thirties, I was experiencing mysterious symptoms and reactions which not even I could understand.

I was walking an emotional tightrope, never knowing when I would stay steady or when I might slip. My reactions were real, and beyond my ability to control. They came out of nowhere. I was very happy with the real me, but the fake me was a disaster.

Clearly my lifelong allergies began in infancy and have continued to keep me company throughout the years in varying degrees. Looking back, the progression makes sense, and no matter where you are in your life's journey, my discoveries will most surely allow you to find encouragement and comfort here. If we had known then what we know now, my life story would have taken a much different turn.

Childhood
#earlyillnessandantibioticsalerttheallergicmarch

In 1951 my parents and I moved from Cleveland, Tennessee, where I was born on Ocoee Street, to Oak Ridge, Tennessee, where my father took a job with Union Carbide Corporation at the nuclear weapons facility. We often returned to Cleveland for weekends with our large Hardwick family, whom I adored.

We stayed with my grandmother on Centenary Avenue but sometimes I got to spend the night with my beloved great aunt, Mary Walker Parks. She lived in one of the older Cleveland homes on Worth Street, and it was a very special place. On summer evenings we would sit out on the front porch in the wicker swing or in the large green rocking chairs and eat homemade peach ice cream while we watched and talked to the neighbors until bedtime.

I always slept in the special guest bedroom with Ace, her beloved cocker spaniel, close by my side. On cold evenings the well-stoked coals glowed all night in the sculptured wood fireplace and in warm weather the tall windows were kept open as the organdy ruffled Priscilla curtains fluttered gently in the breeze. Intricately carved antique furniture topped with beautiful pink Tennessee marble gleamed softly in the moonlight. The imaginary chubby faces in the Cabbage Rose wallpaper were not scary. I loved that beautiful old Victorian pattern. As a young child, sleeping in the ornately elegant authentic

Lincoln Bed made me feel valued and important. The musty old Oz books, so carefully chosen earlier that day at the Cleveland public library (located in an old Victorian home on historic Ocoee Street) were carefully tucked away beside me. I loved them so, but I would get drowsy and fall asleep long before I could finish reading them. Next time, I would check them out again. The goose-feather pillows and soft down-filled blue satin coverlet made me feel so warm and cuddly, like a pampered princess.

After a favorite supper of ground beef patty, creamed rice, sweet green peas, toast with real butter and Aunt Lula's homemade pear preserves, what little five year-old girl wouldn't just float away into a heavenly sleep...

Aunt Mary always smelled so sweet, a soft mixture of Pond's Cold Cream and White Shoulders cologne. I loved her with all my heart.

So why did I so often wake up sobbing in the middle of the night? I had no idea what I was crying about. No bad dreams that I could remember. I wasn't homesick. I loved the chance to "sleep over" on Saturday nights. Everyone seemed worried, and determined to come up with a solution. I felt awful when Aunt Mary would say, "Oh my precious darling girl, what is making you cry?" I felt such a strong need to give her an answer, but I couldn't. I didn't know. What if she thought I didn't love her? We needed an answer. We didn't have one.

Adults in the family tried to help, but even at my very young age, their solutions made no sense to me.

"She's scared of the wallpaper."

"She's homesick."

"She has a stomach ache."

"She's afraid she'll get a stomach ache."

"She's heard stories of Lincoln and John Wilkes Booth."

"Somebody hurt her feelings."

"She just doesn't like it there. Maybe she shouldn't spend the night..."

No telling what they came up with among themselves but didn't tell me. I was so afraid I was hurting Aunt Mary's feelings. I just wanted to stop crying in my sleep. The first mysterious scenario had reared its ugly head.

I loved attending services at Broad Street Methodist Church. Everyone gathered downstairs for an old-fashioned early morning sing-along before Sunday school. It was exciting and joyful and I loved being with so many family members and friends. But so often I had to stay home, especially after an overnight at Aunt Mary's. I would awaken with my top lip so swollen I could barely speak, much less sing. It felt as if I had been given a huge injection of novacaine. Today you could equate it to a giant dose of Botox, gone terribly awry. Again the adults, trying to help, offered their explanations.

"She ate too many helpings of something."

"An insect bit her lip."

"Too many strawberries."

"Maybe it was the chocolate."

"Hot dogs are not healthy."

"She must have eaten something that didn't agree with her."

As if I had done something wrong. Now if that were the case, why didn't someone explain what it was so I wouldn't do it the next time? Why didn't it happen at home? No one knew, of course. I just wanted to solve the mystery. It made Aunt Mary sad, but she always knew how much I loved her. It made me sad too. I was like the princess and the pea, only the tiny pea was totally illusive and could not be found.

I was 40 years old before I finally began to understand these childhood mysteries.

My middle childhood years were uneventful for the most part. My parents were heavy smokers and our house had no air conditioning in the 1950's, which meant the windows were open most of the time. East Tennessee air was humid and we lived in a wooded neighborhood. We had puppies in the house, but they were not allowed to sleep in our beds. Mold and pollen flowed freely and abundantly most of the time.

In first grade, 1953-54, I missed 167 days of school. I had measles, mumps, scarlet fever, whooping cough, tonsillitis, bronchitis, mumps, chicken pox, allergies, impetigo, and asthma. If it could be caught, I caught it. But still, I made straight A's and was reasonably healthy in between frequent doses of antibiotics. Penicillin was out of the question, so various sulfa drugs and other medicines were tried in an effort to accomplish the appropriate antibiotic remedy. Both my tonsils and my adenoids were removed, but neither of these surgeries seemed to make a difference in the trail of recurring illnesses throughout my early years. Later I was told my tonsils were growing back.

My mother was a great cook and there was never a lot of junk food in the house. Fast food restaurants had not yet arrived on the scene, and my classmates and I ate the same cafeteria lunches at school every day. In third grade I weighed 108 pounds and was the tallest in my class. I decided to go on a diet. One night I wanted only vegetables, and ate three helpings of green beans. It made sense to me at the time. My parents thought I probably shouldn't have three helpings of anything. I was confused, wanting to lose a few pounds but not knowing how. My daddy, who was slender his entire life would say, "Eat the fat, it's good for you." I resisted his advice, but judging by what nutritionists are advising us today, he might have been on to something. Then later, he would tell me to watch the starches. At my cousin's house, her mother made homemade mayonnaise and spread it on saltine crackers for our snack. She started to hand me one, and then took it back. "Oh, I forgot," she said. "You are on a diet." I wasn't given anything at all. She wasn't being mean; she just didn't understand. And neither did I. Another mystery in need of solving.

I never grew taller than 5 ft.2 in., and through childhood, my weight fluctuated but I was generally in the normal range, a little pudgy at times but I don't remember anyone ever commenting on it. Seasonal allergies began to appear, and asthma interfered with outdoor activities, sports, and dance lessons, even when I wasn't really sick. "She will probably outgrow it," they said. I didn't.

When I was five years old, I wanted to be a ballerina. Mama bought me leotards, tutus, tap shoes, toe shoes, and a pretty pink ribbon for my hair. Ballet lessons were held in a beautiful musty old building with shiny polished oak floors and floor-to-ceiling mirrors. The smooth wooden barres smelled like furniture oil and our beautiful teacher reminded me of magnolia blossoms. I loved every minute of it. That is, until I got sick. As soon as I stepped into the classroom, coughing and wheezing took over. It made dancing too difficult and although no one ever said so, I am sure I must have been a distraction to the other young aspiring ballerinas and our instructor. Needless to say, the lessons had to be given up, and my ballet-dancing dreams disappeared. It made that little girl very sad, and until I began this quest, I never really understood what was happening.

As young girls often do, we loved to brush and style each other's hair. That is, I liked to comb other girls' hair, but I did not like for anyone to touch mine. I remember Aunt Lula bribing me to let her brush out my curls. She was the only one with a patient tender touch, and she offered me a nickel for every time a tangle hurt me. Nickels meant a lot back then. A few years ago a friend and I were reminiscing about those wonderful early years. She asked me why I never let her brush my hair and why I was so tender-headed. I just smiled and told her she would have to wait and read my book. Now she knows.

In junior high school, I dreaded gym class because we had to run laps and I would get so out of breath. Once I passed out on the hot cinder track, trying to run the 440. It was my asthma. "You'll be okay," my teacher said, "just take a few deep breaths." I didn't feel okay, and I couldn't take deep breaths. I was trying not to cry. I wanted to be athletic, and there didn't seem to be any concern about why this was happening to me. At the time it was not considered very important for girls to play sports or be athletic. My symptoms relating to such things as wheezing, low energy, shortness of breath, headaches, and temporary flu-like symptoms were inconsistent and variable. It was not as if I passed out on a daily basis, so apparently there was no real cause for alarm. I always wondered why I often reacted differently from most of my friends, but I didn't dwell on it at that age. The next reaction would probably re-incarnate itself. It might present as something entirely different, like sleeping for two hours as soon as I got home from

18

school even though there had been no strenuous activity and I had slept well the night before. Another mystery. "She's just tired," they would say. "Young girls need their beauty sleep."

I was extremely allergic to cats. My friends didn't believe me, even though I would cough and wheeze and my eyes would water and my back would itch and I would have a general case of "the miseries" whenever a cat came near me. They were certain it was because of something else, and wanted to prove it. In the ninth grade we went to a friend's house and I was sitting on the sofa. Two girls kept me occupied, while two others sneaked a large tabby into the room and hid behind us. Within a minute I became congested, and the other symptoms quickly followed suit. From then on, my friends understood a lot more and the cat mystery was solved. Still I wondered, why did this happen? My friends gave me a sterling silver cat to put on my charm bracelet to commemorate the event and show their support. I cherish it still. It means a lot because it signifies that they believed me and no longer thought I was just making it up. Through this whole process, validation has been important. Allergy symptoms are real, and cats will sneak their way in and out of my story as we go along.

All through high school I continued to have bouts with allergies and asthma, but my quality of life was fine. There was the usual bronchitis every spring, every fall, and sometimes in-between, but regimens of various antibiotics usually cleared it up within a few weeks.

I always cried easily, but there was nothing in my happy childhood to make me sad. My life was fun and exciting and I was loved and respected. No tragedy, no home problems, not even boyfriend problems. My friends often told me I should go on stage and become a movie star, because it was so easy for me to cry. I was probably one of the happiest, most well-adjusted girls in school, but sadness and tears would suddenly appear at the oddest moments. "Tollie is depressed," they would say. "Let's go to Shoney's and cheer her up with strawberry pie!"

Foreign languages and journalism were my favorite subjects in high school. Senior year I wrote a column for the local newspaper entitled, "Teen Talk Topics." I only had to visit the printing facility once a week to turn in my column and I never wanted to stay there very long. When they offered me a full time summer job I turned it down. For some reason I didn't feel my best inside the building but I never understood why.

Once for a project I contacted ten of the largest newspapers from around the country, requesting a weekend copy of their papers. I remember sitting on my big bed, surrounded by all this newsprint. Couldn't wait to get started, but I was so drowsy. I couldn't keep my eyes open, and fell sound asleep. Mama said I slept for 4 hours that afternoon. They didn't wake me up, assuming I had been up late too many nights studying. Why was I so awake and anxious to get started one minute, and overwhelmingly lethargic the next? I didn't understand it, but something was bothering me and it had to do with those papers. No one believed me. It was a mystery, but now I know.

Sophomore year in high school I started getting headaches on a fairly regular basis. My family doctor found no medical explanation and thought it might be my eyes. Regular school eyesight screenings were always normal. I was devastated when I failed the eye exam when applying for my driver's license. Coming home without that coveted piece of paper is every teenager's nightmare. When I arrived for my test that Saturday morning my eyes were swollen and red. It turns out I had been up all night at a "slumber" party the night before, at a friend's house. Their home could have been full of unknown allergens. At this point, there is no way to evaluate the situation. At any rate, I passed the second attempt with flying colors.

COLLEGE DAYS
#allergicinfirmaryhoursimpedescholasticsuccess

In 1965, I went off to college at the University of North Carolina at Greensboro. I soon lost some weight, down from 125 to 110 pounds, but I didn't understand how it happened. I ate at the school cafeteria, and was not on a diet. My family assumed I was not eating right and occasionally I spent a week or so in the infirmary. My energy was good and cafeteria food was healthy and delicious.

My two roommates smoked cigarettes freshman year, and before long I tried one too (it helps you stay awake to study, they said) and it was very stylish at the time. I was immediately hooked. Looking back, I think I was probably already addicted to nicotine, from breathing the second-hand smoke always present around my parents. But if so, why has my younger brother never smoked? Maybe he never tried. Maybe it is the allergy factor that makes the difference. Siblings don't always react the same way. We probably will never know. I gave up cigarettes a few years later. It was one of the hardest things I ever had to do.

I wrote for the school newspaper my freshman year, but I was always much happier out in the field interviewing for stories and writing them in my dorm room than I was in the printing press area. I understand that now.

I enjoyed Biology my sophomore year until one morning in early October. I went to my lab station and there on the table was a huge dead cat, waiting to be dissected. I almost lost my breakfast, but managed to stay long enough to read our instructions. I was coughing and wheezing and disrupting the class and soon found myself being escorted out of the laboratory by my professor. I don't even remember walking back to the dorm. It was a huge lab, and there must have been as many as twenty cats on the tables. It seemed like at least a hundred.

We know now that avoidance is the best medicine, but this is a perfect example of how you cannot always avoid surprises. I managed to pass biology, but it was the only D I ever saw on a report card. Another mystery: maybe it would have been an A if we had dissected frogs instead! I ended up in the infirmary for a week. As usual, my congestion quickly turned to bronchitis, and I was back on the antibiotic regimen, trying to manage the infection as well as the heightened asthma symptoms. I guess the cat allergens combined with musty autumn leaves and everything else proved to be too much for my immune system. A second round of antibiotics ensued, but I never heard a doctor or a nurse mention the word allergy. With such a violent reaction, why didn't anyone even discuss the possibility of prevention? It puzzles me still.

One spring after a trip home, my cousin offered to drive me back to school on his way back to Washington and Lee University in Lexington, Virginia. He drove an old Corvair, and fumes poured into the front seat area through the glove compartment. No problem, he assured me, we would just leave the windows rolled down. Our trip took eight hours through the winding mountain roads through Boone, North Carolina and on into Greensboro. We didn't stop to eat. Mama had packed us a lunch basket of sandwiches, Cokes, brownies, and bananas. By the time I made it into my dormitory room, my room-mates said my skin was actually green, and I immediately passed out on my bed. Being college students, they assumed I had been drinking so they took care of me as if that were the case. I assume the smell of those black fumes mimicked alcohol so their assumption was logical. I don't know what a severe hangover feels like, but it could not be worse than that. By Monday morning studying was hopeless and I missed two days of classes. I had no fever or other specific symptoms but it felt like a severe case of the flu and I doubted if I could ever get back to myself again. I cried a lot, but never understood why.

Junior year I transferred to the University of Tennessee. My room was in a very clean, air conditioned high-rise dormitory and my energy levels were at the highest point I could remember. I began to put on a little weight, and before long I was sleeping every afternoon when my classes were over. Walking up and down the hills to get to class was becoming more and more of a challenge, and my asthma overwhelmed me at times. I found myself looking for classes that were easier to get to, at the bottom of the hill. We didn't drive cars to class back then. It was a struggle.

Marriage and Children
**#itwasnoaccidentmefindingyousomeonehadahandinitlongbefore-
weeverknew**

After college, I married Michael DeGraw in a beautiful ceremony at Broad Street Methodist Church in Cleveland, Tennessee. I weighed

106 pounds, less than I had weighed in the third grade. It was a storybook wedding in February. The temperature was 7 degrees. We left the next morning on a plane bound for Honolulu, Hawaii, where we lived near his family for a couple of wonderful years.

I felt good there most of the time, but headaches were frequent, and sometimes the only way to relieve them was to go to sleep. Aspirin had little or no effect. The headaches would come and go, sometimes very slight and sometimes excruciating. Because they were not constant, no diagnosis was ever made and I just learned to deal with it. The climate agreed with me and trade winds were amazing. They kept the humidity low and mold spores at a minimum. The tropical climate was also low in pollen.

As a newlywed I got along beautifully with Michael's family. We lived with them for a while and the only complaint my mother-in-law ever had was about the vacuum cleaner. I was always happy to help around the house, but she once complained to Michael that I never cleaned the vacuum and put it away neatly when I was finished. It was my least favorite chore. It was probably all I could do to stuff it back into the closet and go take a nap! I always dreaded vacuuming. It made me feel sick, but I had no idea why. It was a mystery at the time, but now I know that all that dust and pollen being sucked in by the vacuum cleaner was spewing those monsters through the cloth bag and right back into my face.

When we returned to East Tennessee I soon became pregnant with our first child. At that time expectant mothers were told to always "eat for two" and neither the doctor nor my family was concerned about weight gain. I was still smoking, and no one suggested it might hurt the baby. My friend's doctor suggested that smoking might reduce the size of the baby a little bit, and she reasoned that giving birth to a small baby wasn't such a bad idea, the more she thought about it. By the time I was eight months pregnant, I weighed 186 pounds. I was always out of breath, and my allergy symptoms were becoming worse. The mold count was very high that early spring, and as my ankles began to swell, my condition became more severe. I had to take an early leave of absence from my job at the Nuclear Safety Information Center. I just couldn't cope.

My doctor put me in the hospital on a very strict diet. I had toxemia, a severe condition characterized by high blood pressure, swelling of the hands, feet and face, and excessive protein in the urine. The causes are still not clearly understood. Dietary deficiencies are suspected which brings food allergy to mind, and I am most certain that general allergies played a part as well. I was only eating iceberg lettuce, canned tuna, and a little cottage cheese every day. Hot tea was okay and lots of water. I did not lose weight. I started crying. The lady in the bed next to me tried to help by talking to me and she was very nice, but I honestly could not say what was making me cry. The nurses tried to comfort me, assuming I was scared and worried about both the baby and myself. They didn't know anything about my family and thought maybe I or someone else was blaming me for not taking care of myself. They must have wondered, considering the fact that the tears continued to flow.

Nothing was further from the truth. Michael and my family loved me unconditionally. They treated me like a queen and I was sure the baby was fine. I had one of the best obstetricians in the country. He was kind and competent. We were all doing the best we could. Still, I was sad and the more people quizzed me about why I was crying, the more frustrated I became, and the more I wept. I didn't have an answer and no one was helping me find one. It was the happiest time of my life, yet those aggravating bouts of sadness would not leave me alone. Why? Another mystery.

I went home from the hospital but two weeks later I was back again, and this time they induced labor. It was a long, tedious 28-hour process and we were all exhausted. Michael never left my side and the doctor was monitoring me constantly. They had to give me lots of medication and I don't remember the birth. I finally woke up several hours later and I cried again (happy, explainable tears this time) to hear that our beautiful baby boy was strong and healthy, waiting to meet his mother. My swollen ankles began to shrink and my blood pressure was returning to normal. I still had asthma and allergy symptoms to deal with, but there were no other complications to baby or me. It took a few weeks for my energy to return and baby was on formula, because that is what the hospital gave us at the time. No one ever even asked if I wanted to nurse our baby boy. Prepared formula was touted as the preferred choice for all modern consumers back then, without question. There was no known (or publicized) connection between breast feeding and allergy prevention for babies during those years. Thankfully scientific research is finally beginning to find a link between pregnancy, breastfeeding and allergy prevention, but it is in the early stages and nothing definitive has been proven.

I still needed to lose about fifty pounds so my family doctor prescribed diet pills, which were legal amphetamines, commonly prescribed at the time. My weight gradually returned to about 120.

A couple of weeks after Andy's birth, we were living in an apartment and I started feeling uncomfortable. I would have crying episodes but nothing was going on to cause the sadness. It was a joyful time in my life. These sad tears were puzzling but now I remember that every month the apartment was sprayed with a smelly product as part of their pest control. The chemical fumes remained in the air for a long time. It was annoying but we never considered it to be a health issue. By the time the early seventies rolled around, cloth diapers were obsolete. Disposable diapers were all the rage among new parents. I read somewhere that in 1970 American babies went through 350,000 tons of them. Each was infused with a soft "baby-fresh scent." My mother once mentioned that she missed the true and natural scent of tiny babies. That seemed odd to me at the time, but now I know I would have been much better off without the fake fragrance.

I was frustrated because everyone, including my doctor, brushed off my symptoms. They attributed it to the fact that I was overwhelmed with the responsibilities of being a new mother. They were wrong. I knew my feelings were not normal. It was not post-partum depression because it was not constant. One minute I was laughing and happy, then I would become anxious or tearful. I had plenty of help and support, Michael and I were so much in love, and the baby was perfect. Why was I feeling so anxious and depressed one minute, and fine the next? Why did I cry? I was offended by my doctor's mere mention of the vague term "Baby Blues." This tiny new baby was the joy of my life. It was yet another mystery, begging for a solution.

When Baby Andy developed a rash, his pediatrician suggested that I had used too much soap in the laundry or maybe it was the bleach. He diagnosed it as skin allergy and prescribed Kenelog cream. Overall, the baby was healthy and happy. He slept well and woke up smiling. He did, however, get the sniffles a lot, and was diagnosed with allergic rhinitis. For many years, orange-flavored Triaminic syrup was his constant companion. We didn't think much about it, and he was a healthy baby except for occasional minor inconvenient allergic episodes. Growing up, he was smart, popular, athletic, and a natural leader. He missed very few days of school.

Andy loved baseball from an early age. When he began to play ball, I noticed a disconnect between his desire to practice and excel and his actual follow-through. It was inconsistent but his desire and love of the sport never wavered. His natural abilities served him well and he played baseball in college but I always felt that there was a missing link. His size could have been a factor. He had trouble gaining weight, but I truly believe he had what it took to play in the Big Show. Why it didn't happen has always been a mystery to me. As his mother, I knew him better than anyone. He thrived in the hottest summer days on the ball field, but in the Spring and fall he seemed to have a hard time waking up in the mornings, and if he fell asleep during the day, he would wake up, sometimes a couple of hours later, groggy and irritable. He could be moody for no reason and was easily frustrated, yet we all got along fine and there were no significant problems.

One fall he and his dad set up a sock with a baseball in it hanging from a tree branch in the edge of the woods in our back yard. Andy wrote up his practice schedule and posted it on his bedroom door. He was eager to swing at least 100 swings every day and he would strengthen his wrists by driving long nails into a large cedar log. Moldy piles of wet autumn leaves surrounded his perimeter and soon his enthusiasm waned, and the schedule was forgotten. It could not have been a change of heart. He was not lazy. Something happened. It was a mystery. He was having trouble with his nose, possibly a deviated septum from sports, and his eyes were excessively dry. Triaminic Syrup, his constant "cold remedy," was no longer working. We took him to the local allergist who suggested surgery for the nose and tests to diagnose the allergy symptoms.

The test came back negative, and the doctor said he was not allergic. This made no sense to me. He was diagnosed with allergic rhinitis as a baby and I did not believe he had ever outgrown it. This was really a mystery. If my allergic state had been better controlled I feel certain I would have been more persistent, but I was too allergified and my personal knowledge was limited at the time. We reluctantly accepted the allergist's test results.

In the meantime, I had found Dr. Pienkowski. I gave him Andy's brief history and my thoughts about his health. He immediately explained that there was such a thing as a false negative test result. He tested Andy and the results were astounding. He was highly allergic to all molds, trees, grasses, pollen, animal dander, and so forth. He had food allergy as well. He was allergic to potatoes, tomatoes, corn, mushrooms, milk, and more. All the things teenagers loved to eat. Was it good news or bad news? Time would tell. He certainly didn't fit the definition of a wimpy kid with allergies. Far from it. Yet still, as a young man, he was reluctant to accept the results.

Andy was scouted and invited to try out for an elite baseball team in Cincinnati and went for several days to a camp at Xavier University. He excelled beyond anyone's expectations, including his own. Different air, clean new air-conditioned facilities, sports nutrition and other factors helped him immensely, in my opinion. He decided not to accept their invitation to join the team, but I always wondered what life might have offered him if allergy were not a factor. It remained a mystery, but I was beginning to find the clues.

It is important to note that false negatives do occur. If it happens to you and something doesn't seem right, never hesitate to question the results. These things do happen and it is always wise to get a second opinion. Or another allergist.

Michael's job took us to Des Moines, Iowa in 1972. I became pregnant and took a job as bank teller. I loved working with the public, and even though math was never my strong suit, working the register and balancing out at the end of the day were not difficult tasks. That is, until I began to get drowsy and had difficulty focusing. By the end of the day I almost always had a headache. I had to close my eyes for a few minutes at lunch time and on breaks. I worried that I might go so sound asleep that someone would have to wake me up. I wondered why I became so drowsy when I was not tired and had plenty of sleep the night before. I soon found that I had to run several tapes at the end of the day to balance my station. I could not seem to get through without input errors.

Simple tasks became tedious frustrations and I could not understand what was going on. This simple math was becoming more irritating than my college trigonometry course. Michael and I finally decided it was because of my pregnancy. Hormones or something. My asthma and other sneezy-style allergy symptoms were no worse than usual, and I was always much better once I got home. The dry Iowa air agreed with me. I resigned my job with much regret. Once more, Michael was faced with the full financial responsibility and more than his share of duties on the home front.

Our second child, baby girl Jennifer, was born in the middle of a huge Iowa blizzard. My pregnancy had gone well, and I only gained 40 pounds this time. When it came time to deliver, we went by taxi in the middle of the night through blinding snow to an unknown hospital where my doctor was stranded. I remember watching *Jeopardy* while in labor and cheering on a contestant who was a friend of mine from college days. This pregnancy was easier than the first one. This is often true, but I believe a lot had to do with my environment. My allergies had been out of control in the humid pollen-infested April spring when Andy was born in Tennessee. On the other hand, mold and pollen are totally insignificant, even non-existent, in a January Iowa snowstorm. My allergic condition at the time was probably close to the same thing as being immunized, but we were clueless back then. My doctor came in and grabbed my hands. He said, "We are short-staffed because of the blizzard and there is not an anesthesiologist available. We have to do this the natural way." I was not prepared and I had no idea what he meant. It turned out to be good news. Baby Jennifer came quickly.

Without the after-effects of heavy medications and anesthesia to deal with, I felt wonderful. I had a slight headache, which turned out to be caffeine withdrawal. It went away easily with my first cup of coffee. Again, no one asked if I would be breast feeding; they just brought the formula which was assumed to be the best choice for all babies. I suppose the formula manufacturers had a lot to do with that, and at the time we were still unaware of the benefits of breast feeding for the baby's immune system. Current research indicates that breastfeeding may also help defend children against the development of food allergy.

On the way home from the hospital I asked Michael to stop at the Mall so I could pick up a few things. What a difference this was. Why was I cheerfully shopping, two days after this birth, and in bed for two weeks after the first one? More mysterious questions, going unanswered for a long time, but now we know.

From Des Moines we moved to Winston-Salem, North Carolina. Baby Jennifer developed a rash all over her body, and I was told I used too much bleach in her laundry and caused her to have an allergic reaction. Apparently it was my fault, as if I should have somehow known better. I wondered why none of the rest of us had a problem as our laundry was included with hers. There was no explanation, but to me it was a mystery, and somehow I was to blame. We were there for a short time and except for a minor bladder infection, an erroneous diagnosis of "Sponge Kidney" and a minor related surgery for polyps, my allergy symptoms remained present but manageable.

One afternoon we found a black widow spider under the coffee table right where the children were playing. We took care of it of course and Michael rushed to the store and came back with a huge can of bug spray which we promptly emptied in a cloud of vapor, all around the apartment. Almost immediately, I began wheezing and soon the tears came, and I was so agitated and feeling upset that I could barely function. My head was pounding. After sleeping for hours, I still felt very strange and out of sorts. They thought it was just an emotional reaction, thinking of what could have happened if that deadly spider had bitten our children. I always knew it was much more than that, something out of my control. I just didn't know what and I couldn't prove it.

We moved to Indianapolis, Indiana and together with friends, we planted a huge vegetable garden in their back yard. I tried to help with it, but the smell of fertilizer made me sick and the hot sun made it even worse. I loved the thought of working the land, but it just didn't seem to like me. I tried to help harvest the bush beans, but finally after bending over the rows for a while in the hot sun, I passed out. Such was the end of my gardening that summer. I wondered if it was something about me and green beans, but at that point it was still a mystery. Now I know.

I quit smoking in 1975. Andy came home from kindergarten and told me he did not want me to die so could I please quit? It moved me to tears, and I threw my cigarettes away. Michael was away on business and he had already quit. I cried for three days, trying to stay normal for the children, but I felt nauseated, sick and miserable. It did subside, however, and I was able to break that awful habit for good. My addiction was very strong, but thankfully I never smoked again.

From Indianapolis we moved back home to Oak Ridge. Nearby Knoxville was designated the allergy capital of the country. Mold and pollen hung in the humid air and wreaked havoc with my asthma and other symptoms. Still I wasn't really aware of what was going on and as the seasons changed, so did my symptoms. We were glad to be back with the family, and nothing else mattered. I could handle the at least twice-yearly bouts with chronic bronchitis and the illnesses in between. Being sick to some extent most of the time was becoming second nature to me, and I was good at hiding what was really going on with me emotionally. I did not want my allergies to affect those around me, but avoidance was becoming harder as time went on. The constant medications needed to control my outward symptoms were taking a toll on me. It often seemed that they were worse for my system than the symptoms they were supposed to control. No one, not even my doctor, understood why I felt that way.

Jennifer was happy and healthy as a young child. She complained of stomach aches from time to time and was sensitive and caring towards her friends and family. Tears have always come easily to her, and I believe her hidden allergies remained unnoticed for a long time. She was slender, athletic, musically gifted and a popular leader. She was good-hearted with a terrific sense of humor but negative thoughts would sometimes make her sad. She was always singing and at age ten she was determined to learn to play the piano. We couldn't afford a new one, but we found an old player piano at an estate sale. It was in good tune and we couldn't wait for her to start her lessons. She rushed through her homework in order to have more time to practice.

For some reason, unexplainable at the time, her enthusiasm and energy changed soon after she sat down and began to play. As it turned out, that musty old piano was actually moldy on the inside. I had carefully bleached and polished the exterior, but now we know that all those felt pads were harboring mold. Every strike of a key spewed allergy-inducing mold spores into the air.

She also wasn't happy with her piano teacher, and I suspect cologne and scented candles in her home were to blame. Jennifer finally gave up her dream of playing piano, and it makes me sad to know she regrets it still today.

As a young adult Jennifer was lead singer in several bands. A Nashville studio musician once told us that she could be the next Karen Carpenter. I have to admit that I believe allergy played a large part in the fact that a professional career was not in our daughter's future. She loves to share her voice with those she loves, but was never motivated, dedicated, or energized enough to take it to the next level. Today she takes her allergy shots regularly, under the guidance of Dr. Pienkowski, and is a loving healthy, daughter, mother and friend. We are blessed to have her nearby. As eager as I am to blame so many things on the allergy connection, part of me feels relieved that we don't have to share her with a worldwide stage.

THE FLOWER SHOP YEARS
Oldagecreepupshouldnotbegininthethirddecadeoflife

We never really felt connected to Indianapolis. I now suspect that the unavoidable allergens associated with life in a large industrial city were more than partly to blame. When an opportunity presented itself in 1976, we were happy to move back to Tennessee. My parents were considering buying Price Florist, where my mother had worked for many years. The current owners were retiring, and their historic business, among the first developed in what was then called the Atomic City, was for sale. They wanted to keep the traditions of their successful contributions to the community in good hands, and our family was poised to take over. In 1976, Michael and I went to work there, eager to learn the ropes, considering a partnership if the opportunity worked out for all of us. I absolutely loved designing the floral arrangements and working with brides and special occasions. Michael was learning the business side and his background in sales and marketing as well as his gift for working with the public made it a natural fit.

My first words of advice: If you have allergies, do not go to work in a flower shop!

Mama had often complained about dreading the Easter holidays when the lilies came in. They made her sneeze, and their pollen was everywhere. The spring season was short however, and no flags went up warning me to beware of the allergy factor for myself. The floral environment didn't cause me to sniffle and sneeze to any great extent, but before long I began to feel overwhelmed.

At first I convinced myself that it was simply adjusting to the hours, the responsibility, and taking care of two young children while holding down a full-time job. I was smart, other women were managing their own businesses and raising families successfully, and I was certain I could handle the task. There were many more unusual obstacles in my way, but I was not yet aware of them. Actually, the flowers themselves were not the biggest monsters in the shop. It was pollen-covered Christmas greenery, scented pinecones and artificial trees, newspaper ads and wedding write-ups, silk flowers and dried material, aerosol cans of Green-Glo plant polish, cash register receipts, potpourri, daily bookwork, spray paint, scented candles, colorful catalogues and consumer fragrances, just to name a few.

We eventually owned two flower shops and I see now that even though we were exceptionally successful from a business standpoint, my health was deteriorating. Michael was taking on more and more responsibilities, both with the business and our personal lives. It was all I could do to keep up with the design work, weddings, and special occasions. I was very good at hiding my problems, because I did so want us to be successful, but the odds were not in my favor.

In the early days when allergens were still in control, I was feeling old beyond my years. Old age creep-up should not begin in the third decade of life. In my sixties I felt like I was still in my thirties. Not as I actually felt in my thirties but how I think I should have felt. Back in my thirties it often seemed as if I were in my eighties, suffering the unwelcome effects of deteriorating muscle, bone, and brain. I was always tired. My joints ached. My muscles were sore. Everything took extra effort and everything was a big deal. Getting to work was a struggle. Getting home from work was a struggle. I remember at times saying to myself, "You can do this, just put one foot in front of the other." My parents had more energy than I did.

It was the age of the emerging woman. Stories on the news and in all the magazines were touting the successful lives of modern women as they skillfully and happily managed their families and their careers.

I had a good brain and all the blessings and support anyone could hope for. I should have been at the top of my game, but sometimes I felt as if I were about to hit rock bottom. Looking back, I call this time in my life The Geritol Years. Back then, in the late 1970's Geritol was advertised to the older generation as a tonic guaranteed to diminish the inevitable signs of aging. Every dose was supposed to represent a visit to the Fountain of Youth. It was not designed for someone in her thirties, but I was desperate, and I gave it a try. Sadly, it made no difference. The term "wise beyond her years" is a compliment. "Old beyond her years" is not. I was fighting a losing battle.

At the end of a long day working at the flower shop (which I loved), I wanted to go home, cook a nice dinner, play with the children, help with homework, plan the next day, and snuggle on the sofa with my husband. I truly believe I could have done it if the allergy factor had not been so severe and so unrecognized. I could do it today.

It is important to note that I was not on a downward spiral. There was no consistency and there were plenty of good days. Usually if you have a disease, it is constant or it continues to become worse. With me there was no progression, and complaints to my family doctor (without any specific symptoms such as bronchitis) resulted in a diagnosis of "You are just working too hard. You need to get more rest." That, of course, was not the answer. My symptoms floated in and out from day to day and week to week. I didn't fit into any specific category. Allergy and environmental issues were not understood, and I wonder at this rate if they ever will be. I hope I am helping to raise consciousness about the possibilities and the urgent need for research, compassion, and thinking outside the box.

Never once were there any complaints from Michael or the children. They thought I was caught up in the "Super Mom" syndrome, but it was so much more than that. I wanted to be one of the mothers in the magazine articles who was always smiling and in control, but instead I felt more like I belonged in the Geritol commercial. No matter if you are in your thirties or your sixties, if you are feeling tired, achy and overwhelmed without explanation, please consider consulting an allergist. If he only wants to treat your sneezes and sniffles, I suggest you find another allergist. It could save your life.

From my first conversations with Dr. Pienkowski, I began to realize that I had chosen the wrong career. His dedication to healing people as opposed to treating symptoms was evident from the beginning. Rather than immediately insisting that I give up my association with the flower shop, he took the time to educate me slowly so that I understood everything that was involved in my healing. I remember saying at one point, "So I have to give it up?" And in the kindest way possible, he answered, "Yes." He could have simply agreed to prescribe medicines to treat my symptoms, but that is not who he is.

As the years went by, our house became less and less healthy. We were so busy and overwhelmed that we were becoming less aware of the details than we should have been. We found ourselves delaying even basic chores if they were not absolutely necessary at the time. Unknown to us, there was a small leak under the house causing the crawl space to become damp, and that became a breeding ground for mold. Not the dangerous toxic kind, but just a high concentration of everyday mold spores, the ones to which so many of us are allergic. The patio flooded and leaked inside to a concrete floor which was covered with indoor/outdoor carpet. We thought all the water was removed, but we were misinformed. The still-damp padding beneath the carpet became a perfect environment for more mold and bacteria. We couldn't see it, and we didn't smell it for a very long time. We were all becoming allergified but since everyone responded in their own way, the big picture was clouded, and we did not make the allergy connection for years.

When it became time to make repairs, we decided to include some additional remodeling. It was a disaster. Since it was winter, almost all the repairs were done inside. There was sawdust everywhere and nothing was covered properly. Carpet was pulled up and left for days, leaving us to breathe even more of the musty air from the padding underneath. The plumbing vent pipes were installed incorrectly, creating a sewage gas problem. The construction crew jack-hammered the concrete patio floor to improve water drainage and the fine cement dust floated through the inside air. By the time we realized we had to move to a hotel, everyone was sick and I was a basket case. I was reluctant to leave home, not trusting the workmen to do things correctly, but I was too sick to stay there. I was so upset about the whole situation that I was becoming part of the problem. My immune system was a mess so everything turned into an infection. Once again, Michael was left with more than his share of the responsibilities, but he never complained. I complained enough for both of us.

We ended up hiring a prominent Knoxville law firm to force the contractor to make things right. Our attorney kept telling me, "This is not a health issue." We ended up in court. Now I know it really was a health issue, and I regret not forcing the court to look at it from that point of view. Today my brain would let me argue the points in an intellectual way, but it was a mystery back then. I could have made a difference for others who faced similar situations, but it was not to be. My intelligence was controlled by monsters, and I just gave in.

The jury apparently believed that this was an insurance issue and we were double-dipping the system. Nothing could be farther from the truth. They held no one responsible and awarded the defendant one dollar for his troubles. I was devastated. The law firm apologized for not educating the jury properly and waived all fees. It was never about the money.

Even after the city inspectors were satisfied that everything was safe and up to code, we were still not safe. Mold, saw dust, cement dust, paint, and varnish, among who knows what other contaminants lingered in the air we breathed, and my symptoms continued to escalate.

I am convinced that these events contributed greatly to my severe allergic disease. The best possible outcome, other than an eventually healthy home, is that it set me on the path which led me straight to Dr. Pienkowski's office in Knoxville, Tennessee.

After saying good-bye to the flower shops, I needed something to do. I knew I was too sick to handle a full-time stressful commitment as

I began the healing process. Michael and I agreed that a part-time job which allowed me to be home with the children in the afternoons and during the summer holiday would be the best idea. In the late 1980's I took a job as classroom assistant in the local Montessori school.

To those of you who are not familiar with the concept, Montessori education was developed by Italian physician Maria Montessori in the late 1800's. It is a child-centered approach to learning in which children ages 2 ½-6 work together in one classroom using specialized materials developed by Dr. Montessori. Children move freely (within reason) guided by their individual instincts throughout the clean, quiet, orderly prepared environment. We used all-natural products and foods whenever possible as they were considered best for the health and safety of the children. It was a novel concept at the time.

Now I know that the hours I spent in this pristine environment were healthy and safe for me as well. Our only classroom pets were goldfish and young children don't wear perfume! I can say with confidence that our monster-free environment helped me get well.

Even though the paychecks were not large, I was able to contribute financially, and the job was perfect for me. Before long the school board began encouraging me to pursue the rigorous training and develop a classroom of my own. Intellectually, I longed to say yes, but I just wasn't well enough to make the commitment. I resisted their urging, offering various excuses, for a very long time, even when they offered to pay for my degree. There was no way I could explain what was going on. I barely understood it myself. I excelled at my job, and although allergies were always present, they were fairly quiet in my classroom, and I hardly ever sneezed.

As my treatments began to show results, I attended training sessions and teaching workshops in places like Atlanta and Orlando. Traffic and new environments were both mentally and physically challenging. I was often drowsy and lethargic, but I managed and I fought the monsters as best I could.

St. Nicholas Montessori School of London offered a correspondence course (no internet back then) and I finally agreed to give it a try. I studied at home during the summer with a personal tutor/mentor. I was successful only because I could choose to work when my brain was clear. I finally attained my master's degree from Memphis State, thanks in part to my air purifier, the amazing Bionaire 500, which ran constantly in my dorm room.

I loved my work at Montessori, and various stories relating to my students appear throughout this book. A large part of my training involved extensive observation skills which I credit with helping me uncover the clues needed in my own recovery. One of my favorite quotations comes from Maria Montessori. She said,

> "A hundred years from now, nobody will remember
> who I was, what I did ,or how much money I had.
> But the world may be a little different and a little better,
> because I was important in the life of a child."[2]

A healthy environment clearly does make a difference, especially to those of us who are allergic. If we focus on clean surroundings, both indoors and out, and if we really pay attention to what we eat, breathe, touch and smell, we and our children will become much more well-nourished and well-adjusted as time goes by. In addition, we will be helping to prevent a plethora of allergy-related health issues for the next generation. I have great faith in Dr. Montessori's common-sense philosophy. Had it not been for my severe allergic disease, I believe I would have owned my own Montessori School. Clearly that was not God's chosen path for me.

---

2   Dr. Maria Montessori, source unknown

The Healing Process

The Steps to Recovery
TESTING

#itishardtosolveaproblemifyoudon'tknowwhattheproblemisinthefirstplace

I am amazed at how many people are convinced they don't have allergies when just by looking at them I am convinced they probably do. I am also amazed when people complain about their allergies but have no idea what is causing the problem. Many are so used to living with their symptoms they are no longer even curious. And then there are the parents who refuse to have their allergic children tested because "it might hurt." It might hurt the parents, but the children will be just fine.

There are at least two reasons for allergen testing: One from the physician's perspective and the other from that of the patient. From the patient's point of view, it will help eliminate the guesswork, well-meaning random opinions and judgements from others, "old wives' tales," and old-fashioned home remedies which may have worked for others but do not work for him or her. Its purpose is to identify culprits and find peace of mind. The allergist, of course, is looking for facts.

If you only sneeze when you smell tulips in the spring, the answer is self-evident. Avoid tulips. If you self-examine closely and you really are not feeling quite yourself, more is going on behind the scenes. Testing uncovers the whole picture.

If I had not agreed to be tested, I would not be well enough to write this book today. That is a fact.

Once it is determined that a person is allergic, allergy shots are not always recommended. Sometimes avoidance and medications are sufficient. The doctor cannot give a complete diagnosis unless he or she can identify and assess the severity of the offending allergens. Just like in so many different areas of our everyday lives, you cannot defeat the enemy if you cannot even give it a name.

Modern allergy tests are extremely accurate. When the allergist orders a test, his nurse puts little dots of cool wet substances (extracts from food, pollen, mold, dust, etc.) in rows along the patient's back. She then pierces each spot with a tiny little needle. If the word "needle" scares you, feel free to call it a "lancet" instead. Whatever term you use, you will only feel a quick pinch, like getting bitten by a tiny little bug. The entire process takes only a few minutes. The site may itch, and if it turns red you are allergic. After about 20 minutes, the doctor examines each prick and determines the strength of the reaction. If immunizations are indicated, his laboratory prepares the serum formula to coincide with these observations.

Testing is safe, reliable, and relatively painless. Rarely are there any types of adverse reactions. Insurance policies cover testing and serum under the preventive category, so for most people cost should not be a deterrent.

For both my family and me, getting tested for allergens was one of the smartest and most important undertakings we have ever accomplished. I highly recommend a clinical evaluation for anyone with known allergy symptoms and particularly for anyone suffering from unidentified medical mysteries. If like me, many of your symptoms and their causes are intermittent, hidden and unclear, this procedure will go a long way in solving the mysteries which are preventing you from experiencing life to the fullest.

Immunotherapy
#allergyshotsarenotpainfulandfearofneedlesisallinyourhead

The single most important step to my recovery was becoming

immunized. It had to be done. I was allergic to almost everything on the test, including lots of foods. It was a welcome surprise, because then I could identify my enemies and together with Dr. Pienkowski, we began our attack. My successful immunity allowed me to validate personal conditions previously labeled as unexplained or even imaginary.

It soon became clear that leaving the floral industry permanently was our only option. Attaining and maintaining an allergy-free status would always create too much of a challenge while working in that environment, no matter how much I loved it. Dr. Pienkowski helped us understand the far-reaching implications and we soon realized that reducing exposure was a necessary component in my treatment plan. Floral design was no longer in my future. Tot and Tollie's Flower Shop and Queener Flower Shop suddenly ceased to exist. A lucrative on-line worldwide floral delivery service would have to wait for someone else to develop. If only we had known then what we know now.

Like most people, I was apprehensive about getting shots. Needles are not a pleasant subject. I wondered, "Will they work? Will they hurt? Will I be able to keep up with the schedule?" My apprehension soon turned to confidence, and I realize now that this healing process changed my life forever. Allergy shots are not painful, and unless the nurse doesn't wait for the cleansing alcohol to dry, the tiny thin needle prick is seldom even felt. I am often chatting with the nurse and don't even know when she is finished with the injection of the magic serum.

"Piling on" occurs when allergens stack on top of each other like logs in a woodpile, creating layers of symptoms which eventually overwhelm the immune system. In severe cases like mine, these allergens blend together and hide like individual pieces in a newly opened jigsaw puzzle box. Some pieces are easily recognized. Some are not. Only when the identifiable pieces are discovered and removed can the remaining illusive ones ever be found.

For example, if you are sneezing from pollen in the spring, your symptoms may improve with time on their own. If at the same time your family adopts a kitten, you develop poison ivy, you contact a respiratory virus and Aunt Harriet comes to visit wearing her "Jungle Gardenia" perfume, things can get quickly out of hand! Allergy shots prevent piling on by eliminating reactions to most common allergens. Those of us with the remaining food and chemical allergies will then be more able to identify, isolate, and avoid them whenever possible.

Piling on is a complicated concept. One day your symptoms could feel overwhelming, and the next day they could be minimal. Did you ever take a sick child to the doctor only to hear the reply, "I'm fine," when she inquires "How are you feeling today?" This scenario illustrates the illusive nature of the allergic experience.

Most patients do not have much trouble with the initial stage of their treatment. I was different. The first phase of my immunotherapy took longer than usual because of the severity of my condition. My doses increased in tiny increments. Whenever I had a reaction to an injection, they would have to cut back the dosage. Sometimes large red welts the size of a half dollar would appear on my arms at the injection site. At times I felt sick and needed epinephrine. That was not the normal situation, and Dr. P. told me I was one of his most allergic patients. I was so overwhelmed with allergen overload that anything added to my system was bound to be met with resistance.

Dr. Pienkowski's amazing staff encouraged, comforted, and took care of me as I cried, wheezed, coughed and headached my way through the first few weeks. Talking to others in the waiting room and hearing their success stories kept me motivated, and I persevered. Eventually the welts reduced to the size of a dime and then went away altogether. I gradually went from twice weekly injections to once a week, then every two weeks, and finally to a maintenance dose of only one shot per month.

In the beginning, numerous medications were needed in order to treat my various allergic conditions, including asthma. Dr. Pienkowski monitored my progress every step of the way. As my immune system gained strength and my allergies improved, he gradually weaned me off everything except my antihistamine, which is still available although seldom needed any more.

You will probably hear legions of people claim that allergy shots don't work. Statistics prove otherwise. Allergy shots are actually 80 to 90% effective over time. In my observations, often the human factor rather than the serum appears to interfere with its success. A less than effective serum formula is possible. Some allergists use one general formula for all allergic patients. Dr. Pienkowski customizes each formula to match his patient's test results. In my opinion, a "one size fits all" is not the best approach. Patients' reactions are individually different, and the air in California is not the same as the air we breathe in Montana or Tennessee.

Many people tend to get their injections according to their own schedules rather than following the timetable recommended by their doctor. If you decide to just show up when it is convenient because of your hectic schedule, the procedure will be less than successful and it will take much longer. You are teaching your body to change the way it responds to your allergens. The schedule is designed to provide increasing dosages at specific intervals. The term "hap-hazard" does not apply! Many give up too soon, with unrealistic expectations. Instant gratification is not possible in this situation. Your allergic condition did not develop overnight, and it won't go away overnight. If you are patient, you should see real change by the time the next allergy season rolls around. If you stop the immunization process when you first begin feeling better, your symptoms will return.

At one point I was feeling much better, although never as well as I am feeling now. I got careless and lost track of my specific monthly immunization schedule. My lack of focus was a big mistake and I suffered the consequences. Before I knew it, my fierce monsters returned and I was suffering again. I had to get re-tested and start the whole immunization process all over again from the beginning. It was easier the second time, but I had lost ground. This delayed my symptom-free status for a long time, maybe even years. Faithfully following your prescribed schedule will most definitely provide the best results.

If you have an allergic child, I strongly suggest that you have him or her evaluated by an allergist. In certain situations, children can be tested as early as six months. Otherwise there is no age limit. Treating symptoms year after year may work well enough, but in more severe cases, immunization could be the best gift you could ever provide. Immunity unlocks the door to a potentially healthy life and it lasts forever. Don't be fooled when symptoms come on in the spring and get better in the summer. An allergic constitution never goes away. Decongestants cause more problems for children than they do for adults, so it is important not to judge your children's reactions by how they affect you. Many children become hyperactive or drowsy after taking certain antihistamines or other symptom-reducing medications so it is important to notify the teacher if they have been given any of these medicines, even several hours before school. Poor performance could easily be misconstrued.

While sitting in Dr. Pienkowski's waiting room, I often see families with young children go into the injection room. They come out smiling, and very seldom do I hear a child cry. Clearly, children perform better in school, in sports and other activities as well as being less tired and more well-behaved when they are not allergified. Protecting them from these real monsters is even more important than protecting them from the imaginary ones living in their closet or under the bed. I often wonder what my life would have been like if early immunotherapy had been available back in the day.

Another important point to consider is that as adults get older, allergy medications often become problematic. They can interact with blood pressure and other necessary drugs. They could also contribute to asthma, osteoporosis and other side effects. For example, a congested nose and irritated throat could be dangerous to a senior who is suffering from pre-existing cardiovascular problems. First generation antihistamines are very effective in controlling allergy symptoms but have been associated with serious problems such as confusion, sedation, blurred vision, dizziness, and reduced mental alertness in older individuals. Second and third generation antihistamines have fewer side effects, but early immunization for allergic patients seems to me to be the best solution of all. There doesn't appear to be an age limit on receiving allergy shots but as we get older, other diseases and conditions come into play. If a time comes when it is too late to begin an immunization process, "just dealing with it" might become your only option.

Even though Dr. Pienkowski's office is 30 minutes away in Knoxville, we are able to get our allergy shots locally at our family physician's office, which makes it very convenient. Maintenance inoculations are monthly for most people. Whenever a new bottle of serum is needed, a simple phone call to Dr. P's office is all that is needed. It is ready in a week or so and when the temperature is not too hot, it is shipped right to our door.

Michael and I continue to get our shots together every two weeks, just as we always have. We could probably stretch it out a bit but since this is working so well, we see no reason to change anything. Dr. P. concurs. I call his serum my "Liquid Gold."

MEDICATION
#medicinemakesusfeelbetterbutalifelongregimenisnottheonlyanswer

For most of my life I have needed some sort of medication. Because I suffered a life-threatening exposure to penicillin as an infant, an allergic tag has been permanently attached to all my medical records. This began a series of sulfa drugs, antibiotics, cough syrups, lozenges, nasal sprays, pain killers, decongestants, antihistamines, eye drops, bronchial treatments, diuretics, blood pressure meds, asthma medications and inhalers, along with tonsil removal, adenoid removal and even more medicines and treatments I can't even remember.

Beginning in my early teens, I could count on antibiotics at least every fall and every spring as seasonal coughing and congestion eventually turned into bronchitis and sometimes even pleurisy. Similar intermittent episodes occurred throughout the years, always resulting in symptom-reducers and antibiotics. I would be out of school for a couple of weeks each time, and if I was still coughing, teachers would send me home. Clearly I was not contagious, so I guess I was a distraction to the class. I did a lot of studying at home, and fortunately I was a good student. Prevention was never even discussed, so I accepted it and dealt with the situation as best I could. I missed a lot.

In college it was the same pattern. My freshman dorm was a beautiful old wooden building. Mold and asthma went hand-in-hand. The infirmary staff and I were soon on a first-name basis. I felt bad for my roommates who had to put up with my wheezing and coughing, but fortunately they were very understanding. I don't know whether doctors did not know how to prevent these predictable illnesses or whether they were content for me to keep coming back for more visits and prescriptions. Either way, it was frustrating for me and my family, but just a matter-of-fact situation to the physicians. That is, until I met Dr. Pienkowski, some 20 years later.

For years I thought that taking many of my medications made me feel even worse than the illness itself, and as a result, I put off going to the doctor for as long as I could. Over-the-counter medicines designed to provide allergy relief were even worse. I remember one time I took one of those tablets on my way to go grocery shopping. I became drowsy and pulled into a parking lot. I woke up two hours later with a headache and no memory of what happened. Sometimes even the so-called non-drowsy formulas have an adverse effect on me. The mere thought of that experience practically puts me in a coma. I have often wondered if some of these OTC medications could actually be working against the body's natural urge to try and heal itself.

As a teenager I was in the hospital for three days for surgery to remove my four impacted wisdom teeth. The nurses loved to tease me by telling everyone how nervous I had been before the procedure. The truth is that I actually fell asleep and they had to wake me up to give me the pill to relax me before the anesthesia. I had to spend an extra day in the hospital because the effects of medication took so long to wear off sufficiently for me to be released.

Avoiding medication was a futile attempt, because my symptoms never went away of their own accord. Antibiotics, especially erythromycin, made me too tired to get off the couch. It was a helpless feeling and I hated it. It was like being trapped in a tunnel, unable to get out, or swimming in deep water, trying to reach the surface. No one understood. Well-meaning doctors dismissed my complaints, explaining that since I was sick, my body needed the extra rest. I should just give in and "deal with it." I would get better over time. It was more than that, but nobody believed me. Until Dr. Pienkowski. His insights and clear understanding of my situation eventually allowed me to move from a state of over-medication to that of non-medication. Releasing my body from the overload of excessive medical ingredients cleared my head and changed my life.

He listened to my complaints and discovered that I was indeed allergic to erythromycin. My symptoms were not the usual rash or stomach issues, so it had gone undetected. It turns out that our daughter Jennifer is allergic to it as well, but it causes stomach issues for her. He found better medicines for me, preferably uncoated and unflavored, and soon the usual suspects became a thing of the past.

Once in 1994 I went to refill my prescription for an antihistamine and was told that my insurance company would no longer cover it. I went to Dr. Pienkowski to see what the problem was. His receptionist called the company and was told that "the committee decided that allergies are just a nuisance and not really a medical condition." We were fit to be tied. Fortunately, we were able to find an insurance company with a better policy. Lack of coverage for everything I needed would have been a real disaster. The company eventually changed its policy.

In addition to plain aspirin I took white acetaminophen in the 1950's and 1960's to ease my headaches, back pain, sore throats and so forth. Ibuprofen entered the market in the early 1970's and for a while it too was white. When all the manufacturers decided that brown coatings were easier on the stomach, plain white pills were replaced on the shelves with those of many colors. Suddenly medications had to look pretty and be easily identified. Bright pink capsules and other coatings set one manufacturer's product apart from the competition. These enhanced medicines, other than aspirin, soon became my only choice, even when I finally figured out that these color-coated pills were causing my abdomen to swell and my head to ache. This created another problem because uncoated white tablets were practically impossible to find.

Buffered aspirin and enteric aspirin replaced plain white chalky tablets as manufacturers added more and more chemicals "to make it better." Taking too much aspirin caused constipation, even when I could find the uncoated variety so it was not always a good choice either. Just as it is with food allergy, minute amounts of these artificial ingredients caused adverse reactions which were hard to identify. I hated the side effects, but they were better than the pain, so once again, I had to "deal with it." I can occasionally locate the purer form of over-the-counter pain medicine, but it is difficult to find and more expensive. Once again, I find it puzzling that removing the added ingredients makes a product more expensive. Fortunately I seldom have any pain today so my occasional aspirin does not pose a problem.

Heartburn (also referred to as indigestion) is a symptom of acid reflux, which occurs when gastric contents flow backwards from the stomach to the esophagus. Many people complain of this painful condition on a regular basis. It was an intermittent problem for me, again most likely associated with my food allergies. Many people can correct this problem right away with over-the-counter antacids. Because of my problems with the artificial ingredients, pills were a questionable answer for me. I usually just waited as long as it took for the pain to go away.

When I discovered organic raw apple cider vinegar, my heartburn symptoms completely subsided. This product is alkaline rather than acidic like other vinegars; therefore it works to neutralize the acids in the stomach just as commercial antacids do, only without the added synthetic ingredients. Although this home remedy is not clinically tested and proven, the apple cider vinegar has proved helpful and harmless for me. Of course it is always a good idea to consult your personal physician before trying something new, but this natural solution might be worth a try if you are prone to heartburn or acid reflux.

One or two teaspoons in a small glass of water completely stop my pain, almost immediately. A teaspoon of baking soda in a small glass of water is also effective. Fresh mint has one of the highest antioxidant capacities of any food. For thousands of years it has been used to treat upset stomach and acid indigestion. It is easy to grow in your own back yard. Those companies which sell antacids probably don't take the vinegar or mint connection seriously, but I do. Natural versus artificial gets my vote every time whenever the same result is achieved.

In my late forties, a routine visit to my general practitioner (complaining, I am sure, of my usual symptoms) resulted in a rise in my blood pressure. The reading was 135/90. He immediately prescribed medication. In those days we were taught that once you begin to artificially regulate blood pressure, you are on the medication for life. Michael didn't want me to take it, believing that I did not really have a condition warranting a lifetime of medicine, especially considering my experiences with other types of pills. He was concerned, and rightly so. Subsequent tests in this doctor's office confirmed above normal readings, and he finally convinced us that an ongoing regimen of medication was necessary in order to ensure my hypertensive health.

Later on it was interesting that my blood pressure readings in Dr. Pienkowski's office were always normal, 120/80. We assumed the meds were doing their job, but the readings were higher and inconsistent in the family doctor's office. He kept changing my prescription. I consulted Dr. P. each time there was a change in my prescription and he made sure I was on the correct medication for allergic patients, regardless of what the insurance companies were willing to cover. It was expensive and often out-of-pocket but we trusted his judgement.

One day when we were discussing the fact that the readings were different in the two offices, Dr. Pienkowski's nurse made an interesting observation. She was using the large blood pressure cuff, even though the size of my arm did not require it. When I suggested the family doctor's nurse use the same thing, she got a normal reading every time. I took blood pressure medication, possibly unnecessarily, for over 20 years.

Once my immunizations took effect and I felt healthier than ever, I asked Dr. P. if it was ever possible to get off of blood pressure medication. He suggested we give it a try. We began by taking half of a pill for a few weeks. The numbers remained normal. Then we stopped the current medication and took two diuretics for a couple of weeks, then one a day for a few more weeks. My readings never went above 120/80 and were often even lower. I am happy to say that I continue to be completely off of any blood pressure medication.

We may have spent thousands of dollars through the years for a non-existent hypertensive condition, but we will never know for sure. The reading at my last checkup was 118/72. To me this is an amazing story, and Michael remains convinced that I never needed the medicine in the first place. Although allergies do not cause high blood pressure, the frustrations and anxiety involved in these visits could certainly cause a temporary increase in anyone's numbers. The important message here is that for me, a mystery is solved.

Even though allergic rhinitis and other mild allergic diseases are not generally considered major debilitating illnesses, they are responsible for billions of dollars in physicians' services, medications both prescribed and over-the-counter, millions of days of restricted activity, and absenteeism from work and school. An estimated 67 million Americans suffer from allergies, and 300 million people worldwide have asthma.

We treat our symptoms with antihistamines, nasal sprays, corticosteroids, eye drops, cough medicines, ear drops, skin creams, antacids, medicated shampoos, pain pills, inhalers, tissues, laxatives, nutritional supplements and Epi-pens, day after day, season after season, and year after year. When one stops working, we try something new. Histamines released into the body in response to allergens can make us sleepy, hyperactive and inattentive so we gorge on coffee, sugar, soft drinks, and all sorts of caffeine and energy-boosting drinks and supplements. We calm down with sedatives, tranquilizers, and alcohol, and the cycle continues. In my humble opinion, there is no medication on Earth more valuable than the knowledge which surrounds it. Its value increases incrementally as it is shared with others. I no longer take any prescription medicines.

I have suffered for years with what I call "allergic constipation." It appears to be connected with my food allergy, but I have never been able to associate it with a particular food. The subject is not pleasant to discuss, but necessary because it affects so many people. In the early days I would have severe episodes, and I tried every available remedy on the market. Nothing helped on any consistent basis. Sometimes a product even made matters worse. There were occasions when I would have to deal with a painful digestive issue for weeks at a time. It definitely interfered with my desire or ability to work outside the home.

One year my annual blood test showed a slight calcium deficiency. A supplement was advised. I tried every available over-the-counter calcium tablet I could find on the market. Constipation was always the result. I finally found a product at a local health foods store. Its ingredients are simply calcium, organic nettle leaf, stearic acid, silica and cellulose. I can safely take one tablet every other day, and my calcium levels remain normal.

One emergency room visit resulted in a doctor's insistence that I go home and take orange flavored Metamucil. "It works for everyone," she said. It did not work for me. I was desperate. My family doctor prescribed a bottle of green fizzy liquid which they use for surgery preparation. It made me want to beg for surgery of my own. Finally after three doses, there was success, but massive internal scar tissue was an unwelcome result.

I discuss this sensitive subject because there are better answers and no one should have to suffer this way. Further research indicated that flavored milk of magnesia seemed to be the medicine of choice for most patients. The cherry-flavored liquid was the most popular and the biggest seller. Magnesia pills were no help to me at all. Everything seemed to contribute to my problem. Finally, a nurse suggested I try original unflavored milk of magnesia. It worked perfectly and from that moment on, my constipation is completely under control. Liquid magnesia has a chalky taste and it takes some getting used to, but it is so well worth it. To me it is like nectar to the gods. Apparently the flavorings, colorings, and other additives were contributing to my constipation problem. Today I take one small dose at the first hint of a problem, and constipation seldom, if ever, develops. After my age-required colonoscopy a few years ago, the doctor described my results as "Perfect." It is a miracle to me.

I was never comfortable taking vitamins or nutritional supplements of any sort because of the synthetic but necessary ingredients. There was no way to predict how they would affect me and it was easier to avoid the piling on of unknowns. We gave them to our children when they were young, but now the mere thought of chewy liquid-filled candy-coated colorful gummy vitamins makes my skin crawl. Getting nutrition from a healthy diet and letting the candy treats be candy is a much better idea. I know it is not always easy to be confident that we are getting a good balance of nutrients. I am in no way against vitamins or supplements, especially when medically needed. Sifting through the marketing gimmicks to find the best one is difficult.

Most people get "the miseries" once in a while. Television commercials promise to "cure" all the sniffly, sneezy, wheezy, itchy symptoms known to man. I can only imagine what would become of the big pharmaceutical companies if suddenly there was an actual cure for allergies. Try to imagine what it would look like in places like Walgreens and CVS if all the shelves normally filled with allergy-related products were suddenly empty. Or if all the meds that generally flew off the shelves sat there untouched and gathering dust. These imaginary scenarios give me an eerie feeling and yet considering the possibility that empty shelves could someday be the norm also gives me hope.

I am not surprised that research for cures and vaccines is disproportionately under-funded. A cure would kill the goose that lays the golden egg.

JOURNALING
#youthinkyouwillremeberbutitsbesttowriteitdown

As the years went by, there were ups and downs, successes and setbacks, but my journals were full and I did all the research I possibly could. Sometimes I just scribbled notes, words and phrases off the top of my head when I didn't even know what they were doing there in the first place. Even though my notes were fragmented, intermittent, and sometimes hard to decipher, later on it all began to make sense. Gathering information in the days before the internet was difficult. Sadly that is often still the case as separating fact from fiction online is a continuing challenge. When information is connected to advertising, or when sources cannot easily be vetted, suspicions are naturally aroused. My best judgement has proved to be my most reliable device.

Journaling is all about finding patterns. I soon realized that there is an art to keeping track of useful information. My words didn't always produce immediate results, but as I looked back and re-read them over time, significant repetitions emerged which have allowed me to connect the dots in ways that memory alone could never have provided.

If you decide to keep a journal of your own, I suggest that you consider such things as environment, time of day and date, diet, your emotional state, energy level, abdominal swelling, stress level, digestive issues, pain level, and even numbers on the scale. Nothing is insignificant, but you have to decide for yourself what is important and unusual for you. Details matter. I sometimes gained insight by reviewing notes and journal entries from previous years, even decades. Puzzle pieces never seemed to age.

Having grown up and spent most of my life in Oak Ridge, birthplace of the Atomic Bomb, I have naturally questioned whether or not some sort of radioactive exposure could be responsible for my medical mysteries. It was a legitimate concern, but there has been absolutely no indication of any relationship between my health issues and any sort of contamination. No journal entries have ever been disputed and all my tests have been conclusive. Without a doubt, all of my health concerns have been completely related to allergy. Dr. Pienkowski was absolutely correct.

The phrase, "Physician, heal thyself" is good advice. I believe the words "Allergic Person, know thyself" is good advice as well. This modern busy world often keeps us over-extended and convincing ourselves that there is no time in the day for journaling becomes a convenient excuse. If you are in that category but your life is less than it could be, I urge you to reconsider. Sometimes, in order to achieve success, we have to put ourselves first.

Without proper documentation, blaming wrapping paper and greeting cards for negative reactions would seem like science fiction. It wasn't. Some of my most important discoveries didn't come from scientists, friends, family, textbooks, the internet or doctors, even Dr. P. They came from me.

Even the smallest details are important. For example, if you are keeping a food journal, it is not enough to just enter "salad" if you ate lettuce, tomatoes, broccoli, cheese, croutons from a box and store-bought salad dressing. Lettuce from a salad bar could be sprayed with preservatives, but not if prepared at home. The complete list of everything you just ate goes way beyond a few simple ingredients, and they could all end up as important pieces of the puzzle. I never would have known that a certain brand of blue cheese salad dressing gives me a headache if these two things had not been connected numerous times in my journals. Now that I am no longer allergic to mold, blue cheese is not a problem. I still avoid the offending brand because of its unknown additives, but eating it on occasion is not a problem.

Journals don't have to be elaborate. You can easily come up with your own symbols and short hand. Computers make record-keeping of even the tiniest detail easier than ever. Allergists treat our obvious complaints with medicine and immunizations, but they don't follow us around 24/7. For example, doctors won't tell you, "Mrs. Jones if you quit eating limburger cheese with sliced raw elephant garlic for breakfast every morning, you will probably feel better and have more friends." The concept is true of course, but we don't need our family doctor to tell us so. Sometimes a little homegrown logic can go a long way. Hidden symptoms remain unconnected and even unknown unless we figure them out for ourselves. The few minutes spent charting events could be the best part of your day. Recording and re-reading notes and entries can establish cause-and-effect revelations which might otherwise go undetected for a long time. If you want to solve a mystery, you have to keep up with the clues.

So often I hear myself say, "If only I had known back then." Journaling at an early age could have made a difference. Even after I was totally convinced that I understood some particular cause and effect, it was nearly impossible to convince others. There was no evidcence. My journals backed me up when I began hearing the words, "I never heard of that. You ought to write a book."

There is a huge time lapse between when I first considered the book idea and when my allergies finally reached the stage of remission which allowed me to compile my scribbled notes and put pen to paper in some sort of orderly progression. The following snippets outline various issues I have dealt with throughout the years. Inevitably there are overlaps because so often one symptom or reaction intertwines with another, and chronology is difficult. Once again, this testimonial is from my own reading, journaling, experiences and observations, presented from my heart in hopes that I can help raise public awareness as to what it really means to have an allergic constitution. This book is my light at the end of a very, very long tunnel.

Sick House Syndrome
#ihatehouseworkbutiloveacleanhouse

Avoiding the allergens which trigger reactions is the first line of defense for every allergic individual. If avoidance isn't an option, reducing exposure is the next best thing. When we moved back to Tennessee in the 1970's, ours was not a healthy house. We thought it was, but as time went by we discovered we were wrong. There were hidden allergy-producing dangers concealed in unexpected places.

Finding the cleverly camouflaged monsters was a monumental task, even once we became aware of their existence.

As a result of diligent detective work guided by Dr. Pienkowski the opposite is finally true and our home is my sanctuary. What began as a "starter house" has ended up as our "forever home" because once it became healthy, I was afraid to try an unknown environment. Adjusting to different air, different building materials, different furnishings and so forth was a process I would do anything to avoid. The thought of finding hidden monsters after it was too late to change my mind was more than I could handle.

According to the Environmental Protection Agency (EPA)[3], today's indoor air can be twenty to seventy times worse than outdoor air. Over half of newly constructed homes are suffering from some form of "Sick Building Syndrome." Formaldehyde foam pumped in between walls as insulation doesn't always stay put and it "gasses out" into the air. Combined with new carpeting, particle board furniture and cabinets, chemically treated plywood, wall coverings and various glues and adhesives used in new home construction, the result is often unstable air. When chemicals get sprayed into the duct work they are practically impossible to remove.

These conditions can become unhealthy for anyone but even more so for those of us who are allergic. Those who are unaware of their sensitivity to these chemical elements are especially at risk. Homes with attached garages are also a problem for people like me. We park our cars in the tightly sealed garage where lawn mowers, fuels and other chemicals are stored in the surrounding area. We enter the home through the garage, breathing all the concentrated gasoline and other fumes on the way in. This is not a healthy situation for anyone, especially for children and anyone with a weakened immune system. I was never willing to take the chance.

We worked for years to identify and eliminate the allergens in our home, and nothing could make me go through that process a second time, even if it meant moving into a mansion. Of course I might see

---

3   www.epa.gov

things a little differently if that option presented itself today, now that I am immunized!

Basic housework can be an extremely difficult challenge for allergic people. The process itself is complicated. Imagine the following scenario: If you stir up the dust with dry cloths and feather dusters, wipe down the surfaces with scented cleaners, sweep the floors and empty the dustpan, take out the smelly trash and install new sweet-smelling bags, run the unfiltered vacuum cleaner, clean the windows with ammonia, clean the bathrooms with bleach, and infuse the rooms with air-freshening aerosol sprays, electric plug-in fragrances or artificially scented candles, the air you are breathing becomes so polluted that it is practically impossible not to fall victim to the monsters.

If you find yourself stretched out on the sofa, exhausted, wondering why you hate housework, you are not alone. So you put the small things off next time and the task looms larger. The never-ending cycle continues and you begin to make excuses. Certain chores become easy to ignore. No one will notice. I will try to get to it next time. Before you realize what is happening, you are overwhelmed, and your system is on overload. Other members of the family experience similar problems just from breathing the same air, but of course no one realizes what is really going on. Their irritability gets blamed on something more tangible or it gets denied. The cycle continues and the monsters are not held accountable. That is, until they are finally identified. Even then, acknowledging and accepting an allergen's responsibility for creating domestic chaos takes an open mind. This dilemma has absolutely nothing to do with the desire for a clean house. Monsters were in charge. I would not wish this quandary on anyone.

In the early years before I found Dr. Pienkowski, I got to the point where I could not keep up. I was uncomfortable when chores piled up and I became faced with a real disconnect. Michael and the children tried to help, but in my mind providing a beautiful clean home was my responsibility. Sometimes just giving them direction was more than I could handle. I began to avoid my friends and I made excuses to avoid entertaining. Even the children's friends were not always welcome. I was embarrassed.

None of us realized how sick I was, because nothing was consistent, and I was good at hiding what was really going on. The roller coaster of good days and bad days was confusing. Tasks were enthusiastically tackled one day, but often left unfinished and put off until the next. One thing was certain. It had nothing to do with being motivated to do the right thing. Both Michael and I have outgoing personalities and we loved hosting parties and special events. That was evident in our successful wedding business. As time went on, I avoided having company whenever I could. My cousin Cindy helped me with the words. "It just wasn't me."

Dr. Pienkowski understood what was going on. He offered lots of ideas and suggested various products and procedures designed to help improve our environment.

I had heard of the "Leaky Sink Syndrome" and I did not want to fall into that trap. This syndrome supposedly occurs when people expect their medicines to fix something they could actually fix at the source. It is like when a hole in a pipe is spewing out water and you are busy mopping up the water from the floor instead of turning off the water and repairing the pipe. We set out to allergy-proof our home. Anything less was not an option.

The first thing we did was to cover all the mattresses, box springs and bed pillows with allergy-proof encasings to help control the dust mite population. We removed carpeting and discovered beautiful hardwood floors which had been hidden since before we bought the house. We purchased a small electronic room air cleaner, newly available at the time. I moved it from room to room and kept it by my bed each night. It was completely portable and I could even take it with me when we travelled. I noticed a difference within a few days. As the air became cleaner, our days became better. We switched to a hard cover vacuum cleaner with a HEPA filter and allergy bags.

Our cute little Golden Retriever puppy grew into a large shedding dog and eventually we reluctantly agreed that Murdock had to live outside. We replaced the old piano with a more modern keyboard. We removed the indoor/outdoor carpet and scraped off the glued-down padding from the indoor concrete slab. I stenciled and painted the floor which eliminated the need for any more allergen- suscep-tible coverings. The remodeling mistakes were corrected. The clothes dryer was not properly vented so fibers and fumes from detergents and fabric softeners were making their way into the air we breathed. We re-directed the dryer vent to the outside. A small leak in the roof allowed mold spores to thrive until the leaking rain water finally made a mark on the wall which we could see. We replaced the roof.

Overstuffed furniture, throw pillows and plush stuffed animal toys added to the dust-mite population. We removed decorative pillows, exchanged the toys and replaced the large sectional sofa with leather furniture. We installed an underground French drain system which directed water away from the foundation. I became a "bleachaholic" when I discovered how easily Clorox killed the mold and mildew. Window air conditioners also harbored mold and open windows al-lowed pollen to circulate freely. Today's pollen-proof screens were not available back then. From the first cold morning the gas furnace spewed forth all the accumulated dust from the duct work. We even-tually installed an efficient central heat and air system.

Our home is situated on over an acre of land, most of it in the back yard. For years, along with family, friends, and neighbors, we admired the huge stately sycamore tree which shaded us with its long graceful branches and extra-large leaves. We grieved together when it had to be cut down. The children loved it along with the old-fashioned rub-ber tire swing hanging from the strongest branch. Michael and I liked to imagine grandchildren following in their footsteps someday. Those large leaves were messy when they covered the patio in the fall. They stayed wet and moldy and they were prolific. Large puffballs of pol-len covered the deck for a long time in the spring. I had to stay inside until Michael finally cleared it all away. It was a never-ending battle. We finally came to the realization that our beloved sycamore was creating a health hazard and it had to come down. When the final decision was made, I cried for days, but it was the right thing to do. Today we can sit outside on the glider sipping a warm "cuppa somethin'" in the morning or a cool cocktail in the afternoon. The long ago sycamore memories still make me smile.

If all of this sounds overwhelming, you are not alone. These environmental improvements occurred over a long period of time and each one had an increasingly positive effect. The fact that I was more allergic than most and we had more unidentified contributing factors than most puts the whole picture in perspective. For many people, if any one of these single situations is creating an unhealthy obstacle, it can be easily corrected once identified. The process was not so easy for me. My head was swirling around in a bowl of allergy stew.

Little by little, as conditions continued to improve, so did I. We installed ceiling fans throughout the house which we use constantly throughout the year. They keep the air moving continuously through the filters. We later added an approved ozone generator and ionizer. These small machines attack gas molecules and micro-organisms which are a source of odors. Dust is not affected. Ozone generators at safe production levels work well at reducing mold and similar contaminants in the air. Ionization magnetizes dust and other particles in the air and makes them heavy. The air becomes cleaner as particles fall to the floor or other surfaces where they can be wiped up with a damp cloth rather than floating around in the air and ending up in the lungs. We seldom have to dust any more.

Negative ions are oxygen atoms charged with an extra electron. Don't be misled by the word "negative." Their positive effect is scientifically proven. They are said to neutralize free radicals, enhance immune function, purify the blood, revitalize cell metabolism, and balance the autonomic nervous system, promoting deep sleep and healthy digestion. They are prevalent in natural habitats and appear abundantly around waterfalls, on ocean surf at the beach and after thunderstorms. They attach to positively charged particles like pet dander, cigarette smoke, dust, bacteria, pollen and viruses, causing them to become too heavy to remain airborne.

A good rain is supposed to clear the air of pollen. I used to think it washed the pollen off the trees and leaves, but now I know it does even more. One of my favorite memories involves rainy days. As a young teenager I liked nothing better than curling up on the screened-in porch with a bowl of leftover spaghetti and my favorite Nancy Drew mystery book, listening to the raindrops swishing through the leaves in the woods behind our house. Remembering these times always makes me smile.

Early morning showers are popular with lots of people. The hot water and steam are good producers of negative ions, and perhaps these particles contribute to the general sense of well-being experienced by many at the start of day. They have been called a natural anti-depressant and are associated with improved energy levels and focus. Today there are even filters which remove sediment, dirt, chlorine and odors as water flows through the showerhead.

Houseplants can harbor mold, but they can also help to clean the air. Once I was immunized to mold, we brought in a few, just to try. They really help in the small office which has less natural air circulation than the rest of the house. Healthy plants can even absorb formaldehyde, benzene, carbon dioxide and other chemicals from the air without giving out any of their own. Some good examples are spider plants, philodendrons, golden pothos, corn plants and peace lilies. Several inches of aquarium gravel on top of the potting soil keeps it well-drained and dry.

The true transformation came when we installed our new central heat and air system. It changed our Sick House status to Healthy. We chose permanent washable electrostatic filters which have proved to be life-changing. They are far superior to the cheaper disposable filters made with chemically treated paper. We rinse them off about once a month in the inside shower so that no pollen gets in from outside. Electrostatic filters draw room air in with a fan and use static electricity to positively charge dust particles which are then held against layers of wire until they are washed off by the consumer. They really clear the air of all sorts of tiny allergens. The fan runs constantly to ensure the system's maximum efficiency. If it gets turned off accidentally, I begin to notice uneasy symptoms within an hour or so.

High Efficiency Particulate (HEPA) filters were originally classified by the government as top-secret. They were developed by the Atomic Energy Commission to protect soldiers from radioactive particles on the battlefields. During World War II, scientists here in my hometown of Oak Ridge, Tennessee, used HEPA masks to guard against radiation contaminants while working on the Atomic Bomb.

Modern HEPA filters remove at least 99.97 percent of dust, mold, pollen, bacteria and any other airborne particles with a size of .3 microns. This compares to one 300th the diameter of a human hair. HEPA filters became popular in the 1970s and 1980s. Today they are practically a necessity for allergy sufferers. They provide near total efficiency in removing all organisms considered harmful to human beings.

According to the Environmental Protection Agency[4], today's average American breathes in two heaping tablespoons of airborne particles every day. Our bodies have to process them and then discharge them through our organs. The process is even more complicated if they are producing allergy along the way. Even one small inexpensive air filter in every bedroom, where we spend about a third of our lives, can make a huge difference in quality of life.

Unfiltered vacuum cleaners, especially the soft-bag type, simply blow the tiny dust particles back into the air, often right into the face of the one doing the vacuuming. The allergens hang suspended in the air for at least an hour after the task is completed. My vacuum cleaner was a monster, and it is no wonder how much I hated using it and put it off whenever possible. The invention of hard casings and HEPA filter bags has made a huge difference and housework has become so much healthier than ever before. The actual task of vacuuming was never what I hated. I loved to see the resulting clean lines in the carpet. I hated the way vacuuming made me feel afterwards. I always felt sick, but I hardly ever sneezed.

---

4   www.epa.gov

In the beginning I had to wear a heavy duty respirator when doing any housecleaning. I was reluctant at first, because it looked and felt strange. Even though it would have helped with outdoor work like raking leaves, the vanity factor prevented me from appearing in public. It was not a pretty sight, and I sounded like Darth Vader. As time went on, I recognized how valuable this piece of equipment was, and my insecurity was replaced with family humor. Successful treatments soon eliminated the need to wear it so often, but it was helpful in certain situations for a long time. Modern HEPA masks are smaller, lighter, and much easier to use. They really do work.

Even after we installed our whole-house central heat and air system with its state-of-the-art filters I could not part with my original devices. They have served us well for over 20 years.

I am not qualified to recommend any of these specific products, but in my mind anything which keeps me from breathing allergen monsters is a Godsend. Although I live in a de-allergified environment today, I still have to be careful when company comes. Allergens of any kind can hitch a ride but I am prepared and friends are welcome. Even furry friends are welcomed with open arms.

Components of Allergic Disease
ALLERGIC RHINITIS
#hayfeverhasnothingtodowithfeverorhay

Allergic rhinitis is really just a doctor's term for runny nose, watery eyes and congestion. Commonly known as hay fever, allergic rhinitis does not require exposure to hay, and it is rarely accompanied by fever. It can be either seasonal or perennial and millions of adults suffer with this condition every year. It can be complicated by other medical problems such as a deviated septum (broken nose) or nasal polyps.

Many people treat their mild occasional symptoms with over-the-counter medications, but immunotherapy is very successful in providing lifelong relief. I am amused when people suggest that the cure for allergic rhinitis is to avoid the allergens that trigger reactions.

Unless you live in a bubble, how does one avoid the air we breathe? The only way to avoid pollen and mold is to move to someplace like upstate Alaska, Antarctica, or the North Pole.

Actually, allergic rhinitis is a serious matter. When membranes in the nose become irritated by allergy, germs and viruses invade the area, multiply easily, and cause infection. If not treated properly, this infection spreads to the throat, ears, and sinuses. At that point tonsils and adenoids become enlarged and diseased, and fluid builds up in the ears, often resulting in serious otitis media (inflammation of the middle ear).

As a child I suffered for years with allergic rhinitis, but I don't think we called it that. My mother insisted she was allergic to goldenrod. When the pretty flowers appeared in late summer, I loved to bring her armloads of large bouquets which I gathered from around the neighborhood. Not wanting to hurt my feelings, she talked about how much she loved to decorate the porch, and placed the vase on a table in the far corner outside. The truth is that the flowers could have been inside on the coffee table. Goldenrod is only guilty by association. The real culprit which bothers so many of us is its companion, ragweed. It has the same blooming period, late summer until frost.

Even though many people do believe they are allergic to flowers, most allergens come from trees, grass and weeds, because their tiny pollen grains are most easily airborne. Flowers are less likely to cause problems because their pollen grains are too heavy to be carried by the wind. That's why nature provides bright colorful flowers to attract hummingbirds and the necessary pollinating bees.

Flower growers, those who ship them and florists who handle them on a daily basis are near the top of the list of those most likely to contact allergic rhinitis. The mere thought of all that yellow pollen on the Easter lilies makes my nose itch. I have the added misfortune of reacting negatively to the wonderful fragrances of hyacinths and tuberoses when they arrive in early spring.

Knoxville rates consistently higher than average for pollen and mold levels. The odds were stacked against me! When Dr. Pienkowsk helped me put these statistics in perspective, the effects of air quality on allergy finally made sense. Allergic rhinitis is much more complicated than just a sneeze or two. I will never forget the wonderful uplifting feeling of opening up boxes of spring flowers like iris, tulips and lilies on cold January mornings in the flower shop. It is too late for me now, but I hope others can be immunized if necessary to enjoy the beauty of God's glory, whether it comes in the form of those first fragrant spring blossoms in a wholesale cardboard box or a bouquet of golden summer flowers clutched in a young girl's hands.

Food Allergy

#Ilovetoeatbuteatingdoesnotloveme

Food allergy often falls into the category of a love/hate relationship. Five percent of adults and eight percent of children suffer from food allergy. It is a very complicated subject. What may be nutritious and delicious to one person may be the exact opposite for another. Many who suffer from food allergy experience either a strong aversion to or a constant insatiable craving for the offending food. Eight simple foods account for 90% of food allergy reactions. The "Allergic Eight," as they are called, are wheat, shellfish, milk, peanut, soy, egg, tree nut and finfish.

My first test showed that I was allergic to a wide variety of foods. The list included such things as apricots, string beans, carrots, egg whites and rice. I tried to avoid every food on my list but at every checkup I continued to have what is called "geographic tongue." Also called benign migratory glossitis, it is a condition which causes harmless tongue patches resembling smooth red islands or in my case a long crevice down the center which I refer to as the grand canyon. The exact cause of this condition is unknown, but Dr. Pienkowski always considers it in assessing my allergic condition, especially as it is connected to ingested foods. The fact that my lips no longer become swollen does not mean I have outgrown my food allergy. Perhaps it just re-invented itself in the form of internal systemic swelling. It is still a huge problem.

Some people experience a strong reaction immediately or a couple of hours after eating foods to which they are allergic. Stomach ache, headache, nausea, vomiting, impaired breathing and hives are common complaints and can be easily attributed to a particular just-eaten food. Peanut allergy is a good example of this. Apparently even one one-thousandth of a peanut, such as the exposure from opening a bag, can cause a reaction. Some people avoid certain foods because "They just don't agree with me." Deniers will encourage us to eat the offending food, insisting that "Surely just this little bit won't hurt you." They are wrong, of course.

Identifying the culprits has always been a mysterious process for me. My first obstacle is the fact that I don't experience any of these obvious indicators, so I have nothing to signal the fact that I have just eaten an offending food. Nothing says to me, "Don't eat that." Before my first allergy test, I had no idea that foods were a problem. The results were a surprise. Food allergy is something that stays with me every day and is an underlying symptom affecting any other health issues which might come my way. I am not alone in this and the number of people who unknowingly suffer from systemic food allergy must be larger than is recognized in statistics today. Since most statistics are taken from medical records, I logically surmise that the numbers could rise significantly when we take into account those who are unaware of their condition and have never been officially diagnosed.

An estimated 15 million Americans suffer from food allergies and the numbers are on the rise. According to FARE (Food Allergy Research and Education)[5] every three minutes, a food allergy sends someone to the emergency room. Each year 200,000 people require emergency care for this condition. As many as 150 to 200 deaths per year are possibly attributed to food allergy but the exact numbers are not available.

Once I knew what they were, I made every effort to avoid the offending foods as part of my total healing process. Along the way I found many examples of hidden foods and I became aware of the

---

5   www.foodallergy.org

relationship of foods within families. For example, coffee and wine may be cleared with egg whites. Carrot extract is often combined with annatto to provide the orange color in cheese, and corn products are everywhere. If you are allergic to latex, you may also be allergic to several cross-related foods such as avocado, kiwi and chestnut. I believe that the primary allergic eight foods have something in common beyond their ability to be highly allergenic. Each in its own way is possibly connected on a secondary level to such things as mold, artificial colorants, metals, chemicals and other additives such as hormones and antibiotics. I discuss more hidden ingredients later in the book.

As I began to learn more about my previously unknown food allergies, more reactions became evident. For example, cooking a pot of pinto beans caused problems such as uneasiness or drowsiness when the fumes combined with the household air. Using a crockpot or the oven for slow cooking of such things helps a lot, now that we know. I have even been known to put the crockpot outside when the weather is good. A pediatrician once insisted to me, "No one is allergic to rice." I guess I am the exception to the rule.

As time went on, I continued to test positive for food allergy even though I did my best to avoid the foods on my list. Nothing seemed to help. My tongue still resembled a map of South America with the Amazon River running through it, and it often had a pale white coating on the surface. Rather than doubt me, imply I was cheating or didn't understand, Dr. Pienkowski stood by me and we figured it out. He tested me several times in a row. When I avoided a certain food my test was negative. As soon as I ate it again, the reaction was positive.

The diagnosis was that I am allergic to everything I eat. If someone has a problem with alcohol, he or she can quit drinking. If the problem is food, abstinence is not an option. It was a real dilemma. My first thought was to eliminate as many unnecessary foods as possible. Simplifying my diet was complicated at first but it is much easier now. I began by avoiding additives and preservatives. My term was "God's packaging." I began to choose things such as a banana in a banana peel rather than orange macaroni from a box. I discovered that the term "natural flavorings" can mean anything, and they do not have to be identified on the label. Eliminating artificial ingredients was fairly easy. If I can't spell it, pronounce it, or picture what it looks like, I try not to eat it.

Rotating foods every five days is an option for someone dealing with only a few offending foods. This allows the food enough time to leave the body before it is re-introduced. I would have to go on a five-day starvation diet to obtain the same results. Not an option for me! Foods continue to affect my ability to attain and maintain my optimum weight, and a swollen abdomen is something I have to put up with off and on, but it doesn't interfere with my general state of good health. That is a blessing.

Foods can also be connected to other allergens. For example, if you are allergic to poison ivy, you may have a problem with mangoes, cashews, and pistachio nuts. You do not have to be allergic to a food to have an adverse reaction to it. Peanuts and tree nuts are associated with mold, and I often wonder if these allergies are worse for people who also have mold allergy.

One of my Montessori children had a severe reaction after returning to class from a doctor's visit. He began turning blue and after we called 911 the paramedics arrived with epinephrine just in time to save his life. Fortunately I knew the signs and alerted them to anaphylaxis so they were prepared. Today my classroom would always be equipped with an Epi-Pen but they were not available back then. We knew the child had a peanut allergy but he hadn't eaten anything at school. After questioning his babysitter, I found out that they had a fast-food lunch on the way back to school from his dental appointment. I called the establishment and sure enough, the French fries were fried in peanut oil.

Both Jennifer and Michael have had unexplained lower backaches from time to time. We made the connection for both of them when their tests revealed a peanut allergy. Now when either of them gets a stiff back, they can clearly relate it to the occasional splurge of a peanut butter and jelly sandwich. One of Jennifer's friends had a similar experience. She was having anger issues and therapy was not helping at all. Her doctor determined that she too was allergic to peanut butter, and eliminating peanuts from her diet cleared up the anger problem permanently.

When eating away from home, you never really know what you are ingesting. To me, if I know ahead of time there may be a problem, I just allow for the possibilities and plan my schedule accordingly. I refuse to let food allergy run my life, but at the same time, I try to make smart choices. Now that my allergy shots are doing their job, I hardly even notice my food allergies any more. If I do become drowsy after a meal, a short cat-nap (nothing to do with real cats, of course) usually restores my energy right away.

I have always been a morning person. I wake up early and my most energetic and creative hours are when I first wake up and before I eat breakfast. Even though it is generally considered a good idea to "break the fast" first thing in the morning, the opposite is true for me. I like to put off breakfast as long as possible. I now believe that since the longest amount of time I go without my food allergens is from my evening meal until breakfast, then logically I am at my best after my longest "fast." There are copious theories concerning the body's circadian rhythm and why some people wake up before the alarm while others hit the snooze button three or four times. When we were young, no one dared even speak to my mother before her first cup of coffee. Dad, on the other hand, was often out on the deck, listening to the birds, before first light. For me, food allergy is the most logical explanation and I credit my early morning energy to one of the few benefits my allergies provide!

ASTHMA

#wheezybreathingisworsethansneezing

The word asthma comes from the Greek word "aazein," meaning to exhale with the mouth open. In his epic Greek poem, "The Iliad," Homer referred to asthma in his description of the siege of

Troy. In modern medical terms, asthma is a chronic inflammatory disease characterized by a narrowing of the airways. Symptoms include shortness of breath, wheezing, chest tightening, and coughing. It is very serious and can be fatal.

As America emerged into the 20th Century, asthma was considered to be a psychosomatic disease. Psychoanalysis and "talking cures" were the accepted treatment. Doctors assumed that childhood trauma or poor emotional regulation were to blame for the bronchial spasms. A child's wheeze was seen as a suppressed cry for his or her mother's attention. They thought people with asthma should be treated for depression. This concept was widespread among the medical community and interfered with research and proper medical treatment until the 1960s when the disease was finally recognized in today's terms and anti-inflammatory medicines began to be prescribed. The stigma associated with the asthmatic condition persevered for quite some time.

The concept of this emotional cause of asthma is unimaginable to me. Now that I am cured (my word), I wouldn't know how to create a wheeze on purpose, no matter how much attention I was seeking. I have tried, and I can't do it! Thank goodness modern science has come such a long way. I understand the relationship between allergic asthma and the overlapping symptoms of depression in ways they could not possibly have understood back then.

According to the CDC (Center for Disease Control)[6] more than 25 million Americans suffer from asthma and the numbers are increasing annually. Thanks to Dr. Pienkowski, I am no longer one of them. Sudden severe asthma attacks affect 44,000 Americans every day. Asthma is responsible for one fourth of all emergency room visits every year. In 2007, 165 children and 3,262 adults died from asthma attacks. For me, asthma, allergy, and anger go hand in hand.

According to the World Health Organization[7], 235 million people worldwide have asthma. It is the most common chronic childhood

---

6   www.cdc.gov
7   www.globalasthmareport.org

disease and it occurs in all countries, regardless of level of development. It is officially listed as an epidemic. The WHO recommends immunotherapy as the primary and most effective treatment for this serious and possibly fatal debilitating disease. I agree.

As a child, asthma ruled my life. I remember the almost constant coughing and wheezing and the panic of struggling for the next breath. My parents would rub my chest with Mentholatum, a smelly concoction of camphor and menthol. I called it MMM, Mama's Mentholatum Medicine, and it smelled terrible. The electric vaporizer filled with Vicks Vapo Rub ran constantly beside my bed. They fed me bitter Horehound candy and Smith Brothers strong black cough drops which turned my tongue and my teeth black. Sometimes they put a footstool next to the stove and I would breathe in the steam from a pot of boiling water as they held a towel over my head to make a tent. I don't know how effective these procedures were, but they were trying their best to help me. At least they didn't send me to a psychiatrist! The modern HEPA-filtered air cleaner on my bedside table today is so much more desirable and really does the job. I sleep like a baby all night long.

Many people are unaware of the fact that the majority of cases regarding asthma, especially in children, are allergy-related. The greatest number of these asthmatics react to dust mites, mold, chemicals, animal dander, smoke, and other allergens. Further research has shown that antibiotics and viral infections in early childhood may increase the risk for developing asthma. Children of mothers who smoke are ten times more likely to develop asthma in their lifetime. This was certainly true in my case.

When a person inhales tobacco smoke, unhealthy substances settle into the moist linings of the airways and can damage the tiny cilia (fine hair-like vibrating structures, resembling eyelashes, on the surface of certain cells) which help sweep away harmful mucous and dust. Inhaling secondhand smoke can be even more harmful because of the substances which burn off of the end of cigars and cigarettes such as tar, carbon monoxide, nicotine and other chemicals. While most of us are aware of the dangers of secondhand smoke, there is another monster involved as well.

Thirdhand smoke is the condition caused when tobacco smoke settles into carpets, drapery, upholstery, vehicles and other areas. The residue builds up on surfaces over time. It remains in the environment even after smoking has stopped. It doesn't go away by simply airing out the rooms. It is especially harmful to young children who spend so much time on the floor and tend to put things in their mouths. Thinking back, I do remember a distinct (not offensive) carpet smell when visiting in different homes in my youth. My friends and I would spend hours on the floor, playing games and watching TV. It must have been even worse when shag carpet became all the rage, but we never connected the smoke to asthma or allergy.

My asthmatic episodes occurred less frequently as I approached my teenage years, but I never felt completely free from the wheezing and shortness of breath until Dr. Pienkowski took control. I really struggled with my asthma in gym class. I especially dreaded running on the hot cinder track around the football field in the spring. Once while attempting the 440, I actually passed out, but all anyone ever said was that I must have over-exerted myself. Once again, as if I had done something wrong. Asthma was responsible of course, but they just didn't understand. Another implication, which I ignored, was that I was just trying to get out of running in the hot sun. At least the coaches didn't refer me to the school psychologist. Now we know.

Asthma continued to follow me into adulthood. It often escalated into infections and chronic bronchitis, producing rounds of antibiotics every spring and every fall. There were no answers and I felt helpless in trying to prevent it. I even developed pleurisy on a few occasions.

Pleurisy is an inflammation of the pleura, the moist double-layered membrane that surrounds the lungs and lines the ribcage. These layers keep your ribs from rubbing up against the chest cavity when you exhale. When the lining is swollen, things like coughing, sneezing and even laughing cause a sharp, stabbing pain. It makes breathing very painful. It is not contagious. Causes such as bacterial infection, pneumonia, viruses, influenza and fungus are accepted today, but the connection to an allergic disposition is not yet understood.

You would think from hearing all of this that I must have led life as some sort of invalid. That was not the case. Between episodes I was fine. But when I was sick, it was severe, and unless you have been in my situation, understanding is practically impossible. The non-preventable, unpredictable, illusive and intermittent illnesses which often accompany asthmatics and other allergic individuals are difficult to explain, even now when there is so much research and information available. My personal mysteries are solved today, and it amazes me how many people still struggle for a valid understanding of what is going on in their lives. Identifying allergic asthma could well be the bridge connecting misery and health for many children and adults. There is no longer any reason to "Just deal with it." Dr. Pienkowski prescribed all the proper and necessary treatments through all the early years, and today I consider myself cured.

The process of becoming asthma-free was a long one. It took perseverance, patience, and a determination, not only to understand, but to overcome the complicated layers of my illness. Asthma is not a disease which can be immediately managed with a pill or a device such as a rescue inhaler. Many factors which have the ability to trigger an asthmatic attack are unusual, mysterious and unexpected. I experienced quite a few of them.

One New Year's Eve, Michael and I went to a dance at one of the big fancy hotels in Knoxville. I wore an elegant spaghetti-strapped black crepe gown with matching shawl and elegant higher-than-usual heels. After midnight, the outside temperature had dropped unexpectedly and it was extremely cold. It was a long uphill walk to our car and valet service was not available. The wind picked up as we began our trek up the hill and pretty soon my chest began to ache. Besides shivering and struggling with the heels, I began fighting for every breath. I began to cry. The more Michael encouraged me, the more upset I became. What was happening? By the time we reached the car, I was a mess. I cried all the way home, feeling as if I were ruining the evening for us, but unable to stop. Michael thought I was upset because I had to walk in the cold and feeling responsible because he should have parked closer or he should have gone to get the car and then come back for me.

The cold always invigorated him, so it was hard to understand. Now we know. Asthma symptoms are exacerbated by cold temperatures and exercise. Breathing through the nose in cold weather warms the air before it enters the lungs. This is not an option for mouth-breathers, and I am almost certain my mouth was wide open. My system was already on allergen overload from the evening's exposures to smoke, cologne, gourmet foods and champagne. I was a prime target for the asthma attack.

I am telling this story to further demonstrate the many ways that allergy affects behavior. Certainly my chest hurt and I was crying and wheezing. The worst part is that I was upset and emotional after a wonderful evening, and I could not explain why. Many of the allergic reactions which might have alerted me did not appear during the evening festivities and for sure I was neither coughing nor sneezing at the time. My allergic symptoms were delayed, and would appear later, probably the next day. If we had been more informed, I would still have experienced the physical discomforts but the huge emotional burden would have been lifted.

I hope that everyone now understands that asthma is not a mental or an emotional disease in and of itself, but the side effects can certainly be misconstrued. What happened to us was not our fault, but had we been more aware of the whole picture, we would have been able to plan and deal with the situation ahead of time and much more effectively. Our special occasions nowadays end with laughter and smiles. Those allergic asthmatic wheezes and tears are a thing of the past.

Going forward, I no longer need any asthma medication, and I have not used an inhaler for years; however, once you have suffered with asthma, the airways remain subject to inflammation. The bronchial tubes may be weakened due to the extreme stress endured over a period of time. Contracting a virus or the flu could trigger a bronchial response. If you have an asthmatic child, I urge you to consider allergy shots. Immunotherapy for allergic asthma can prevent the asthmatic lung damage which could become dangerously problematic later in life.

Almost one third of adults who think they have outgrown their childhood asthma have recurrences in their later years. Untreated asthma can lead to emphysema because continued stretching of the bronchial sacs can enlarge the delicate tissues, causing them to lose elasticity and cease to function. The prevalence of asthma declines with age, but then rises again after age 70. It is often confused with cardiopulmonary disease (COPD). Early immunotherapy can be a big help in providing a good quality of life for our aging population.

Thanks to Dr. Pienkowski's vision, his expertise, and his dedication to treating the entire human condition, I look forward to a healthy, asthma-free future. I take pride in demonstrating my quiet breathing to others who complain to me of their asthma. Every deep breath is inspiring, and I revel in my ability to breathe free.

ANAPHYLACTIC SHOCK

#identifyingallergycansaveyourlife

Since allergic disease is not generally considered to be fatal like pneumonia or cancer, its dangers are often underestimated by the general public. Allergies, however, truly can be deadly. Anaphylaxis is a severe potentially life-threatening allergic reaction. It can appear suddenly with no warning, and it can be fatal. One in every six people who have food allergies has had a documented anaphylactic experience. Sadly, many people who experience an emergency room visit related to allergy fail to carry through with their scheduled follow-up appointment. They are taking their chances and rolling the dice.

According to the Mayo Clinic[8], symptoms of an anaphylactic re-

---

8   www.mayoclinic.org

action include the following:

- Difficulty breathing
- Swelling of the throat and tongue
- Skin reactions including hives and itching, flushed, or pale skin
- A weak, rapid pulse
- Nausea, vomiting and diarrhea
- Dizziness and fainting
- Loss of consciousness

As far as I know, I have not been a victim of anaphylactic shock. There were times during my early desensitizing period when I would require a dose of epinephrine after an unusually strong reaction to an injection, but my symptoms have generally been more systemic and vague in nature. I have experienced violent reactions to specific events, but I was never told that my life was in danger. I often wonder if I was on that trajectory had I never discovered the underlying allergic cause of my illnesses. A few of my early asthmatic attacks produced "get me to the emergency room" situations, but my food allergies have always been more concealed, ongoing, internal and mysterious as opposed to a sudden swelling of the throat or tongue.

I do, however, have personal experience with extreme, life-threatening allergic reactions. The knowledge I have gained as Dr. Pienkowski's patient has helped me in several crisis situations. Our granddaughter Sydney has a severe peanut allergy. One Christmas when she was very young, we were entertaining and one of the neighbors unknowingly gave her a piece of chocolate covered peanut butter candy. She spit it out right away but fell ill immediately and was rushed to the emergency room. That scary episode became a huge incentive for me to share my understanding with others.

Once while we were visiting friends in Indiana, their young son began having trouble breathing. At first he seemed to be choking but the Heimlich maneuver produced no results. They lived out in the country, several miles from the nearest medical facility. His father raced him to the hospital in his Austin-Healy sports car, later telling us he reached a speed of 106 miles per hour. It was too late. His throat closed up and this sweet child died along the way. The medical examiner attributed his death to an allergic reaction to the pineapple and cottage cheese he had just ingested.

As a young adult, my cousin Allen died after eating a fast-food hamburger and French fries. Driving home alone, he sensed a problem and pulled into the nearest fire station where the fire fighters, his close friends, tried everything they could but were unable to save his life. The cause of death was anaphylactic shock. He died not knowing he was allergic.

Even after having experienced my cousin's tragic death, I am amazed by how little interest there was among both friends and family in having themselves and their loved ones tested. Food allergy tends to run in families and is often inherited. One would think that after a family suffers this kind of loss, there would be an urgency to get everyone tested so they would know for sure if they too were at risk. My relatives chose not to take my advice seriously, preferring instead to rely on that roll of the dice.

Today we have Epi-Pens and other injectors which deliver a measured dose of adrenaline by self-injection. They can be life-saving in anaphylactic emergencies, but only if you or someone you know understands their value and has one on hand when the need arises. All too often, it is too late for the patient once the ambulance arrives.

Discoveries, Knowledge, and Insight

The Effects of Allergens in the Environment
CRITTERS, CATS, AND CREATURES
#kittensandpuppiesandskunksohmy

Approximately ten percent of the population is allergic to animals. I'm guessing the numbers are much higher than that because many people have no idea they are allergic, and many just don't want to admit it because it might mean they would have to give up their beloved pets. We all love our furry friends and giving them up is not always necessary. Allergy shots are a much better solution, although avoidance does have its advantage.

Lovable and cute as they may be, cats are by far the worst offenders. For many people, just a brief encounter can cause serious allergic reactions. I wish it were not so, but unfortunately these cat characteristics are here to stay, and we can't just wish them away. The idea that removing the cat from the room or vacuuming the furniture and carpets can prevent exposure is a misconception. Hair length doesn't matter because fur is not the problem. The allergens are shed in saliva, skin secretions, and urine. These protein particles are so tiny they can hang suspended in the air like pollen grains, and are easily inhaled. The particles are sticky and can cling to surfaces such as walls, furniture, ceilings, bedding and draperies. They can remain in the house six months after a cat has been removed, and it can take as long as five years for cat allergens in a mattress to return to normal. An invitation to "come on over, we'll put the cat outside," is well-intentioned, but not helpful. Attempts to breed non-allergenic cats have so far been unsuccessful.

My cat allergies, part of life since my early childhood, continued to plague me until my immunizations began to work. Of course we never had cats in our home. The slightest exposure, like petting a cute little kitten in the park triggered my asthma, and once these allergic reactions have started, they are very hard to control. Cats are the one thing that always made me sneeze. Today I am totally de-sensitized, and I can be around cats without even knowing they are there. I know my thoughts are purely psychological, but because of a lifelong aversion, I still prefer to enjoy them from a distance.

Several years ago when I was well into my immunization process, I received my follow-up testing. When the time came to discuss my results, Dr. Pienkowski came into the room with an unusual expression on his face. Apparently I had registered 18 in the cat category. This was an abnormally high number, much larger than the twos and threes which normally appeared on my tests. He was concerned. He asked if for some strange reason I had decided to adopt or move in with a cat. It seemed as if, in his kind soft-spoken way, he wondered if I had lost my mind. I responded with an emphatic no, of course not. Not that he didn't believe me, but the puzzled look on his face could not be denied. I was experiencing no congestion, yet these tests are consistently accurate. A genuine medical mystery was at hand.

On the way home, the answer dawned on me. I turned the car around and returned to his office. I realized that we had out-of-town company the previous weekend. She didn't bring them with her but Monica lived eight hours away in a house with six cats. She must have brought the allergens with her on her clothes and luggage and in her car. I had my highest exposure ever, without laying eyes on a single cat!

The most astounding news is that I was symptom-free, and for the first time I realized that my immunizations were completely successful. The allergens were in my system, but my symptoms were completely controlled. Cat dander was no longer the enemy. At that point all I had to do was maintain my status.

Another time, along my path of discovery, I became very sick, as if all my symptoms were ganging up on me at once. We had just installed our central heat and air system. It was supposed to be making me better. I was worried. After a couple of weeks, I could barely get out of bed. Dr. Pienkowski put me back on all my meds, and I felt as if I were going backwards. These feelings added to my emotional distress. The mystery seemed unsolvable. A few days later, when Michael was mowing the yard, he noticed what looked like fluffy black and white fur all around the central air unit. Apparently a family of skunks had taken up residence beside the unit and their allergens were flying throughout the duct work. I guess skunk dander was not part of my serum formula. We had the system professionally cleaned, and before long I was back to normal. What a relief!

When we were first engaged, Michael's grandparents invited me to visit them in Toms River, New Jersey. After visiting for a few days, they planned a special night out for dinner at the Jersey Shore. His grandmother presented me with a beautiful Angora shawl which she had knitted and embroidered, just for me. Heavenly hand-spun Angora wool is softer than cashmere and light as a cloud. As we drove toward the coast, I began to cough, then sniffle, then wheeze. My eyes turned red and began to water. I was "itchy" all over. We naturally assumed I was allergic to "something in the Jersey air." I muddled through the evening, embarrassed but loved. They were very sympathetic and gracious, but I was miserable, feeling as if I had disrupted the evening for everyone. Later, we finally figured it out. Angora wool comes from rabbits, and yes, even sometimes from Angora cats!

If you suspect you might to be allergic to certain pillows or other upholstered furniture, it is probably not the fabric but the filling inside. Vintage furniture in particular could be the problem. Horsehair was highly desirable up through the 1950s for use in chairs, sofas and pillows, both as stuffing and woven into fabric. Straw, kapok, coconut fiber, excelsior (made from fine wood shavings), hog hair, and Spanish moss are also used, even today. Many of these fibers can last 100 years or more, but eventually they begin to turn to powder, which can billow out as allergens and affect the air we breathe. If you are allergic, especially to horses, you should always consider the fact that the stuffing might be making you stuffy!

Some people react to cats by becoming agitated and angry. One of my Montessori students, a sweet five-year-old girl, was becoming more quiet and subdued than usual in school. Her parents were concerned because she (an only child) began acting out at home, showing signs of anger and aggression. We observed no such problems at school, other than increased sniffling and sneezing in the classroom. She was intelligent, attentive, and respectful. The situation was very puzzling. After much discussion and discovery, we came to the conclusion that her problems began when the family adopted two baby kittens. They spent most of their time in the child's bedroom.

Once when she was sent to her room as punishment, she actually threw a kitten across the room. Her parents were distraught, knowing that childhood cruelty to animals could be early warning signs of later delinquency, violence, and even criminal behavior. Imagining this possibility was scary for all of us. We worked together, journaling, talking, and observing. I became convinced she was a highly allergic child. She was happy at school but not at home. There was no tension or issues between the parents or in the home environment to cause distress. Pretty soon it all began to make sense. They found a new home for the kittens, moved her to a different bedroom, and had her tested for allergies. Today the parents still thank me for referring them to Dr. Pienkowski. Her anger issues subsided with her allergy treatments and removal of the cats. Today she is happy and healthy, enjoying life and a successful professional career.

Another student, aged four, began acting out after school, pouting and complaining on the way to her older sister's horseback riding lessons. She did not want to go, and they assumed she was jealous because she was still too young to participate. She was cooperative with the other students in the classroom and was patient when waiting her turn. She did show signs of allergy by rubbing her eyes and tugging at her ears. Sometimes she would suddenly lose concentration. She often complained of a stomach ache after snack, but never got sick. Her parents thought she just wanted attention, but I knew better. They had her tested and sure enough, this sweet little girl wasn't jealous at all. She was allergic to horses and hay.

If you have pets in your home and suspect you are allergic to them, you might be mistaken. It could be the pollen they bring in from outdoors or the cedar shavings in the gerbil cage or even a particular brand of kitty litter. If you are chemically sensitive, you should suspect the flea control collar or perhaps other powders or grooming products used on your pets. Sometimes just a small change in the environment can make a big difference in your family's quality of life. I was surprised to learn that human dander can even cause allergic rashes in dogs and cats.

Most of us cringe at the mere thought of stinging bees, wasps, hornets and yellow jackets, as well as fire ants, spiders, scorpions, and other insects. In general, almost everyone is sensitive to bites and stings, but for the most part they are nothing more than an annoying nuisance. True allergic reactions, though possible, are rare.

According to the CDC (Center for Disease Control), about two million Americans are allergic to bee stings, and bees are actually the deadliest non-human animals in the country. Every year about 100 people die from their stings. Additional information states that this number probably represents an underestimate, since some bee sting deaths are erroneously attributed to heart attack, sunstroke, and other causes.

People who experience a strong allergic reaction to a bee sting have a 30 to 60 percent chance of anaphylaxis the next time they are stung. Multiple stings at one time, which occur when a hive or swarm is disturbed, can even induce a toxic reaction. Adults tend to have stronger reactions than children do. As a young child I loved walking barefoot through the clover. Stepped-on bees do tend to sting the feet, and when that happened, my parents applied a paste of vinegar and baking soda "to make it feel better," and off I would go again, still shoeless. There is no way to know for sure if these early encounters immunized me because as an adult I have not had a sting, but early immunity is clearly possible.

Allergy shots are very effective against bee stings, and if your work or hobbies require you to be outside, immunization is a wise choice. Waiting for the first sting might not be the best idea, especially if you know you are allergic to other things. Access to an epinephrine injector (Epi-pen) should be a high priority for anyone who works around insects. It could save your life.

I have often wondered if strong reactions to insect stings could be exacerbated by the presence of mold spores or pollen on the insect itself. Bee venom plus a grain or two of pollen could be double trouble in the bloodstream of a non-immunized allergic person.

Almost all of us are sensitive to mosquito bites, but to those with severe allergies, resulting symptoms can be serious. Most bites occur at dawn or dusk when the mosquitos are most active. Male mosquitos are harmless, feeding on nectar and water, but the female of the species is out for your blood. She is attracted to scent, exhaled carbon monoxide, and chemicals in the person's sweat. Her intrusion is really more of an injection than a bite, as she inserts her proboscis through the skin to extract her victim's blood. The resulting symptoms, such as red bumps and itching, are not caused by the puncture itself but by a reaction of the body's immune system to proteins in the mosquito's saliva.

Extreme allergic reactions can occur, even causing lymphangitis (an inflammation of the body's lymph system) or a condition known as Skeeter Syndrome. This condition, caused by allergy to the mosquito's saliva is rare but painful. Symptoms include swelling so severe that the victim's limb doubles in size and the eyes are swollen shut. Sometimes the bite will blister and ooze. Asthma, low grade fever, general malaise, and even anaphylactic shock can occur. According to the Mayo Clinic[9], this condition is sometimes mistaken for a secondary bacterial infection brought on by scratching and broken skin.

---

9   www.mayoclinic.org

Babies, toddlers, and senior citizens are most at risk.

As a child, mosquito bites produced large red welts all over my body, but today mosquitos seem to have no interest in me at all. Thankfully, I must have been de-sensitized over time, or maybe I just outgrew the allergy. Maybe all the allergy serum in my system simply repels them!

There are lots of chemical mosquito repellants on the market these days, but I have yet to find one to which I am not allergic. The rest of the family really suffers from these pests the minute they step outside in warm weather, so family outings get complicated. We found two different natural repellants which are very effective and there are recipes you can make from natural ingredients found in your own kitchen. One smells like garlic and may make you want to order pizza, but if you do, you can eat it outside because this treatment really works. You simply spray it around the perimeter, and the mosquitoes won't cross through the barrier.

Spray-on repellants work well for most people. Rather than deet (the active ingredient), it is more likely the fragrance which causes the allergy. The addition of synthetic fragrances makes no sense to me because mosquitoes are attracted to sweet floral scents in the first place. I wonder if it could it be that manufacturers are attracting mosquitoes so the need to repel them remains strong.

Dust mites, tiny little creepy looking creatures, are too small to be seen by the naked eye, but they are often the allergic person's worst nightmare. These microscopic bugs are only one-third of a millimeter long. One millimeter is about the thickness of a credit card. They live in pillows, mattresses, carpets, draperies and stuffed animals. They thrive in dark humid environments. Their diet consists of scales shed from human skin. Their waste products are on the surfaces we touch and in the air we breathe. They are everywhere! Dust itself is not necessarily allergy-producing. The problem is the mites that live in the dust.

Even the cleanest homes have dust mites, and each of them produces 20 waste particles per day. Scientists have identified 14 potential allergens contained in each one of them, many of which are enzymes. Each female lays between 25 and 50 eggs, with a new generation produced every three weeks. Their debris continues to cause problems, even after the dust mites are dead. Freezing kills the mites, but not their offending residue. They cannot survive in humidity below 50%, and hot water, above 130 degrees kills them as well. Dust mites are a major cause of allergy all around the world. Even though dust mites will never be entirely eliminated, there are many effective ways in which their populations can be contained and controlled. I will address this issue and offer helpful suggestions later in the book.

Cockroaches are an unpleasant but necessary subject to discuss, because not only do they carry disease but they can trigger asthma and allergy as well. Children are especially susceptible to these allergens. These icky pests are responsible for causing year-round allergies for thousands of unsuspecting victims every year. The insects' body parts, saliva and waste contaminate the air much like those of dust mites. The best way to control them is to deny them food, water, and shelter. They adapt easily to various environments and are a worldwide problem. Experts believe that if you see just one cockroach, as many as 800 could be hiding out of sight. Boric acid has been used as an insecticide in homes since 1948. When used properly it is inexpensive and highly effective in controlling cockroaches. Pyrethrum is an organic insecticide which is advertised as a healthy alternative to other chemical products. It can be a real problem, however, to people like me who are allergic to chrysanthemums.

LEAVES OF THREE, LET THEM BE
#poisonivylawd'llmakeyouitch

Most Americans know that touching the leaves of plants like poison ivy, oak, and sumac will likely cause the development of an itchy angry rash. There was even a hit song written about it in the 1960s. A large percentage of the population is clinically sensitive to these plants, and they are found all over the world. Poison ivy in particular grows abundantly here in Tennessee. The allergen commonly found in all three of these plants is a resinous oil called urushiol. It is found in all parts of the plant, including roots, stems, leaves, and berries. Even dead leaves and other debris can harbor the resin all year round. It is also found on the skin of mangoes and the shells of pistachios and cashew nuts. Urushiol is very sticky and adheres to just about anything it touches. Reactions can thus be contacted by contaminated objects such as picnic blankets, clothing, gardening gloves, shoes, landscaping tools, steering wheels, and even household pets. It is incredibly concentrated and never dormant. The American Academy of Dermatology[10] estimates that there are up to 50 million cases of urushiol dermatitis reported in the United States every year. Children are taught to identify and avoid these culprits at an early age, especially if they play outside. Young people aged eight to twelve are the most susceptible. Any Scout will tell you, "Leaves of three, let them be."

Some people experience no reaction to their first exposure, leading them to believe they are not allergic. They may then show sensitivity to a successive encounter, and repeated episodes can become increasingly severe. Gestation time can be as long as 10 to 21 days for the first rash to appear, but most people develop symptoms within 48 to 72 hours. The rash usually causes problems for one to two weeks, but it can last for five weeks or more.

Over-the-counter anti-itch medicines like calamine lotion and hydrocortisone creams are big sellers. They should be used carefully, however, because of their potential to cause their own allergic contact dermatitis when absorbed through the skin. There is even a special soap designed to "remove the oily residue" from poison ivy exposure to the skin. Actually any soapy water can remove the oil if used within a short period of time, but most often we are not aware of the exposure in time for washing to be effective. Soapy washcloths can be helpful, but they could pick up the oil and spread it around, making the reaction even worse. Any contaminated clothes should be carefully washed or discarded immediately after use.

One Saturday in the 1970s I was working in the yard, clearing

---

10 www.aad.org

weeds from the base of a large Hickory tree in the early spring. I was determined to pull up the roots before the leaves appeared on the vines. Apparently there were poison ivy vines intermingled with the English ivy, and I was naively working barefoot and without gloves. Monday morning I woke up and noticed a slight itching on my arms and legs. By the time I got to work at the flower shop my face, arms and ankles were bright red and puffy, and my eyes were nearly swollen shut. They rushed me to the emergency room. The bottoms of my feet were itching and soon large blisters popped up on the soles of my feet and between my toes. We didn't make the connection to poison ivy allergy at first because two full days elapsed before the first rash appeared. However, the doctors recognized my symptoms right away.

Rows of tiny bumps lined my arms from elbow to wrist. I was also experiencing headache, nausea, swollen joints and fever. As I remember, I was treated with prednisone, topical corticosteroid cream and antibiotics to help combat the expected rounds of infection. Cool compresses helped a little, but I was in a lot of pain for a long time with flu-like symptoms in addition to the itching and oozing of open wounds. I was out of work for three weeks and wearing shoes was completely out of the question. I had a systemic reaction, a condition which occurs when the urushiol resin penetrates the outer skin and binds with white blood cells, spreading throughout the entire body. The rash can then appear anywhere in the system over a period of several weeks.

This experience reminded me of an episode when I was ten years old. We took a trip to our family cabin, located on the Conasauga, a pristine river which flows near the town of Tennga, on the border between Georgia and Tennessee. We arrived in the early spring, before the leaves appeared on the trees and vines. The men were clearing and tidying up the property. They built a small bonfire along the riverbank. Apparently poison ivy ended up in the fire. He was unaware at the time, but my dad was highly allergic, and when he breathed the smoke, his lungs absorbed the allergens and he began having trouble breathing. We were miles from the nearest hospital and he was in extreme respiratory distress. I overheard the adults say that if they couldn't get there in time he might not make it. That life-threatening event turned out to be one of the scariest times of my life. With no telephone service, it was hours before we knew if he had survived. By the time they reached the emergency room, huge blisters had formed between his fingers, spreading them out like fans. He was working shirtless, and his whole upper body was covered in an angry red rash. It was a close call, but he survived, and eventually regained use of his hands although some scar tissue did remain. This allergic episode was a valuable eye-opening experience for everyone involved, even his doctors.

So you see, poison ivy can be more than an annoying little itch. Each episode is potentially more intense than the one before. You can even be exposed to the oil as it flies through the air from things like lawn mowing and weed whacking. Urushiol resin lasts forever. I once had a reaction when my allergies had caused me to be indoors for weeks. We assumed I must have contacted it by touching Michael's clothing, possibly from the piled-up laundry.

After years of attempts at avoidance, my poison ivy allergy is no longer a problem. Thanks to Dr. Pienkowski, my shots have been completely successful and the dreaded urushiol monster has been annihilated. Yours can be too.

MOLD

#moldymonstersmakememiserable

There has been a lot of publicity in recent years about the deadly effects of toxic mold. It is scary stuff. That is not what we are talking about here. My experience is with the seemingly innocent non-toxic variety of household mold which floats around in the air we breathe every day.

Mold and mildew are fungi which can be any color or group of colors including white, black, brown, green or any fluorescent combination. It shows up on shower curtains, house plants, damp basement walls, automobile air conditioning systems, refrigerator drip pans, and on Christmas trees and the water they stand in, especially when they are no longer taking water. It can also be invisible. We consume it in cheeses, mushrooms, beer and bread. It has proved to be one of my biggest monsters, and tracking down the source has been one of my biggest challenges.

Mold spores seem to be lurking around every corner and to those of us who are allergic it is also scary stuff. Non-toxic mold is a monster in the making. People can have a negative reaction to mold even if they do not test allergic. If you live in a high humidity area, there are mold preventive packets which can be added to cans of paint. It is similar to the mold inhibitors added to bags of shredded cheese. As a living organism, mold can even take hold and begin to grow in human lungs.

Testing positively for mold spore allergy was the first step in solving lots of my mysteries. The second step was figuring out exactly how it affected me. Tracking it down so I could avoid it was third, and then the fourth and most important step was taking the shots which finally allowed me to become non-reactive. After years of hard work, guided by Dr. Pienkowski, I finally accomplished my goals. Tennessee humidity with its over-abundance of mold spores was more than a temporary annoyance for me. Hopefully my discoveries will help you deal with your mold problems much more quickly.

Many scientists now believe that the "Curse of the Egyptian pyramids" is related to mold exposure. Many of the early pyramid explorers died of mysterious circumstances. Now it seems evident that the cause was exposure to mold that had survived for thousands of years in the vaults of the royal tombs. Like I said, it is scary stuff. The process of improving your situation may seem overwhelming at first, but once you are successfully immunized as I have been, mold spores will no longer have any allergic effect on you, hidden or otherwise.

Mold spores appear naturally in the air we breathe unless there is snow on the ground. It is a living, growing organism which prefers high humidity but cannot grow in temperatures below 55 degrees. It is the most widespread living organism on Earth, and it includes thousands of different varieties. It is even more prolific than pollen grains. High humidity and moisture inside a building can cause mold to grow 100 or even 1000 times the normal indoor levels. It is a monster of huge proportions. When segments of our population live and work in moldy environments, their health must surely be at risk. The effects can be devastating over time, especially for those who are allergic.

Hygrometers are now available as small inexpensive instruments which monitor humidity levels (water-vapor content) in the atmosphere. They are very accurate and will alert you if there is excessive moisture (and the resulting mold problem) in your home. I often notice that dark shady houses can tend to portray the most neglected appearances. Dense vegetation around the outer walls often hides traces of mildew. Mold is often responsible for personal lack of motivation and energy, and these conditions can transfer indoors to the occupants. Sometimes clearing away this damp foliage and debris can make a difference in the health and well-being of those who reside inside.

Occupations which expose workers to higher than average levels include farmers, gardeners, bakers, brewers, carpenters, mill workers, upholsterers, paperhangers, and as in my case, florists.

Now that I am immune to these tiny little monsters, all their overwhelming effects on my life (including asthma) have truly disappeared. No more sadness, lethargy, depression and tears from musty old antique stores spoil my fun, and I can read old books without falling asleep after the first few pages. Blue cheese salad dressing and my favorite deep fried mushroom appetizers no longer spoil an evening out. Raking autumn leaves is much less overwhelming these days, and I don't become agitated singing around an old player piano.

One of the biggest obstacles I came across in my sleuthing is the fact that my major mold reactions often occurred about 24 hours after exposure. Journaling helped me to eventually realize that allergen encounters do not always produce immediate reactions. Recognizing this pattern helped me look back and figure out the exact source of my altered emotional state. Had a mold exposure produced, for example, an immediate sneezing episode, or sudden unexpected feelings of sadness, I could have made the connection much sooner. To be clear, sometimes mold exposure did produce an immediate response, especially regarding my asthma. Inconsistency increased my confusion and delayed my understanding of how it all works, but now I know.

When I began to pay attention to the mold count in the weather forecast, I realized that often my moods would rise and fall with the daily reports. When you factor in the high mold count connected with the constant dampness in our house, the vision becomes even more complicated because the allergens were piling on top of each other every day.

Through these stories, I hope I have opened your eyes to a few possible unexpected reactions I have attributed to mold exposure. Your experiences may be entirely different. Many who test positive to mold react with only the usual allergic congestion, but being aware of the hidden and illusive behavioral connections I have uncovered may provide you with a whole new realm of possible explanations for your unusual symptoms and experiences. There is an answer, and living with moldy monsters is definitely not your only option.

Sun Allergy
#sunshineonmyshouldersmakesmebumpy

Sun allergy, though rare, is real. I never had acne as a teenager. Good complexion genes, I guess. But in the summer I would get flare-ups of what I called "sun bumps" on my shoulders and upper arms. We spent many long hours boating and water-skiing at the lake and swimming in our huge Oak Ridge city pool. As far as I know, none of my friends had the same condition, but maybe the sun connection was not yet established back then.

This rash would come and go on its own, similar yet different from a traditional sunburn. Splotchy red patches and bumps which looked like pimples would appear unexpectedly on my upper arms, but rarely on my face, legs, or other parts of my body. It cleared up on its own after a few days. It didn't itch and wasn't painful, but for a teenaged girl, it was embarrassing. These sun bumps seldom appear any more, but then I am not out in the hot sun for hours at a time as I was in my youth.

My family doctor asked if the affected area was painful or sore to the touch. He suggested that maybe it was the baby oil, iodine, lemon juice or lotion we used to help increase our tans or produce highlights in our hair. There was no sunscreen back then so I don't know if it would have helped. The doctor determined that since the bumpy rash went away on its own at some point, there was nothing he could do. He basically ignored the problem from then on. His suggestions made no sense to me because we used oil on our legs, lower arms, and faces as well, not just on our shoulders. These bumps remained a mystery to me until Dr. Pienkowski told me about sun allergy.

Otherwise known as polymorphic light eruption, tiny bumps and itchy skin can appear one to four days after sun exposure. Also called sun poisoning, photosensitivity, photodermatitis, or photoallergy, it is an immune system reaction to sunlight. Scientists and allergists don't know exactly why some people develop a sun allergy and others do not, but it is possibly an inherited condition. There is no cure.

Those pesky bumps were never troublesome enough to keep me out of the sun, but they were puzzling nonetheless and it is comforting to finally have the answer. Symptoms of sun allergy usually begin in the late teen years. For me, it was a little younger. It is estimated that around 15 percent of the U.S. population is affected. Repeated exposure causes a person to become less sensitive to sunlight and the rash then becomes less severe by summer's end. The desensitization process, called "hardening," usually lasts through the summer, but the bumps can then return at full intensity the following spring. This pattern of disappearance and reappearance affected me for several years.

The sun produces invisible ultraviolet rays that can damage the skin and possibly lead to skin cancer. We all know this. But to an allergic person it is more than that. Ultraviolet radiation causes changes in the skin's proteins. The immune system misidentifies these proteins as harmful and attacks them, producing rash and other symptoms. Some medications, such as acne products, antidepressants, antibiotics (especially tetracycline), diuretics, and birth control pills can increase sensitivity. Sunscreen products are helpful, but they can cause allergic reactions as well. I am better off avoiding the application of chemicals to my skin, especially the fragrant ones, so I choose the shade whenever possible.

Even though those signature bumps seem to be a thing of the past, sometimes small red scaly patches still appear if I am in the direct sun for an extended period of time. Other symptoms are more pronounced, such as headache, light-headedness, lethargy, and even nausea. I subscribe to the wise philosophy, "All things in moderation." In the matter of sun allergy, it serves me well. I try to be outside in the early morning or evening hours, avoiding the most intense sunlight between 10 a.m. and 2 p.m. I have a beloved collection of wide-brimmed hats which I wear all summer. Michael calls me his "hat lady."

Now that I finally understand what is going on, I can easily ignore all those who believe that being allergic to the sun is a crazy concept. I was further comforted when Dr. Pienkowski pointed to his slightly red nose and said, "I have it too."

Camping
#whetherglampingorcampingpleaseforgetthemosquitopunk

From early summers at our cabin on the Conasauga River to camping trips with our young children and Michael's family, I have always loved the outdoors. I loved the damp musty smell of the forests, the woodsy campfire smoke, the moldy autumn leaves, the emerging foliage and flowers in the spring and the hot summer sun, but they did not love me. Looking back, my family probably thought I didn't want to be there. The opposite was true. The joy of planning and looking forward to these outings quickly diminished as my changing environment took its toll. These excursions were among the best times of my life, so why did I get so moody, tired, and unwilling or unable to participate in all the activities? I tried to cover up my feelings, not wanting to put a damper on all the fun, but something just wasn't right. Blaming everything on the fact that I was overweight was an easy excuse, but clearly something else was going on. Making the allergy connection was difficult at first, because as always, I hardly ever sneezed.

I remember one time relaxing in a lounge chair deep in the woods on the edge of the Pigeon River. I loved the gurgles and swirls as the water danced across the beautiful smooth river rocks. The rhododendrons were blooming and there was just a slight nip in the air. The others had gone on a hike but I stayed behind, making some sort of excuse. Before long, my lethargy gave way to sadness and there I was, tears flowing down my cheeks in that beautiful peaceful setting. The fact that I couldn't explain what was happening to me made me even more depressed. I just wanted to be alone.

Campfire smoke was also a problem back then. The fact that I was allergic to Oak, Maple, Hickory, and Cedar trees among others assured that burning logs were bound to be a problem. Asthma, coughing, and other symptoms were exacerbated when I breathed the smoke. The only thing worse than raking leaves was burning them. Nothing was more fun than singing around the campfire, but my asthma, coughing, and other symptoms were unavoidable as I breathed the smoke so I just moved back out of the way and let the others do the singing. Today burning natural logs, pinecones and yard debris in the campfire doesn't bother me, but I still have problems with the chemically treated, paper-wrapped logs you buy at the store, treated lumber, newsprint, and other printed material when added to the fire. If the saying is true that smoke follows beauty, I will gladly put on my ugly face.

For some reason, gas grills are not a problem for me, even though propane is a strong chemical. Charcoal is okay too, once it is burning slowly. Lighter fluid, however, is a real monster. It gets me every time.

Charcoal pre-treated with chemicals is even worse. For us, electric starters are a much better option.

For family outings, I always took along a big pot of white beans and ham which simmered all day in a kettle on the campfire. It was my father-in-law's favorite. Now I know that white beans are one of my strongest food allergies and those cooking fumes cause real problems for me. The only way I can safely cook them at home is if I put my crockpot outside on the patio. Eating them does not have the same effect, and they are delicious. Years ago I read a newspaper article about a young girl who lost her life from breathing the fumes from a pot of simmering Great Northern beans. She died of anaphylaxis. It is never too late to count our blessings.

Two of my life's worst enemies in the camping days were mosquito punk and citronella candles. The strong-smelling citronella speaks for itself. Punk is a flat spiral coil resembling incense which is made from a dried paste of pyrethrum powder. It is suspended on a small stand and the smoldering coil releases fumes which chase away or kill the mosquitoes. The chemicals in the air which chased away the insects made the other campers happy, but they had the reverse effect on me. A mosquito bite was nothing compared to the misery of breathing the repellants. We never understood how to manage the situation back then, but now we know.

Now that I am de-sensitized, I long for picnics and camping trips. The mere thought of being out in nature brings me joy, and I must admit I wish I could have a do-over for when our children were young. I missed a lot and I could have given a lot more, but only I know what that truly means. Mother Nature and I can finally meet on a level playing field.

On special occasions, the family often enjoyed setting off a large fireworks display. As soon as the festivities began, all I remember is holding my breath and running for cover. Last Fourth of July our grandson Joshua brought beautiful fireworks to set off in our back yard. I was like a kid in a candy store, enjoying every minute and never wanting that beautiful evening to come to an end.

Summer nights are magical to me now as I watch the moon and stars reflect and shimmer on the water. No longer do I have to sit alone inside the air-conditioned camper, watching the synchronized dance of the fireflies through a cold glass window pane. If I want to, I can even go outside and dance along with them in the moonlight. All is well.

The Trouble with Travel
#vacationsarevexatiousforallergicfamilymembers

Traveling to unknown destinations has always intrigued me, but travel can be difficult for allergic people. The sniffles and itches can usually be controlled with the proper medication, but when environmental issues affect your energy and your outlook, happy times can quickly turn to not so happy ones.

Obviously, changes in food, water and air quality play a role in how we feel. Sometimes for the better, and sometimes for the worse. Pollen counts are low at the beach, but mold tends to be high. Cold mountain air curtails mold, but evergreen pollen is a problem for lots of people. The chemicals in tap water vary from place to place and we can never really be sure of ingredients when someone else prepares the food. These manageable changes can affect anyone, whether or not they are allergic; but for people like me, travel presents its own unique set of problems. Immunization makes it easier for me to cope but the travel monsters are still an ongoing problem.

Fortunately Michael likes to drive because I am not very reliable as his relief if he needs a break. I call my condition DWA, driving while allergified. I can't predict ahead of time when DWA might appear. Sometimes I can drive long distances, no problem. Sometimes I can't. I have to determine ahead of time if I am "drivable" or "not drivable," depending upon how many monsters are riding along in the car beside me. The terms "drowsy driving" and even "drunk driving" are accurate descriptions of the DWA condition. It is a safety issue, and cannot be wished away. Some people open the car windows to let in fresh air to energize them. This is not always a good solution for allergic people when the air is loaded with pollen and diesel fuel. It could just make the situation worse.

We always turn the controls to recirculate the inside air, but sometimes there is a need to bring in fresh oxygen. Once I yawned 53 times in a row, but I wasn't sleepy. I just couldn't quit yawning. "Car drowsies" are "allergic drowsies" for me, and a change of air or a short break is usually helpful. It can be a real nuisance because having to stop more often than usual does interfere with the destination schedule. Nowadays there are air purifiers for cars and some are even built in, but nothing like that was available in the early years.

Hot coffee served in Styrofoam, paper or plastic cups makes me feel uncomfortable and I began avoiding it in the car altogether until Michael came up with the perfect solution. He makes sure I always keep a porcelain or ceramic mug in the car, available for transferring any hot liquids into a safe, non-outgassing container. Now I can enjoy delicious hot beverages on all our road trips. It might seem like a small thing, but it is special to me.

Hotels are still a problem. Just opening the door to a room and smelling that telltale super-sweet fragrance can lead to emotional upheaval. We have been told that the spray is used so that the supervisor can determine whether or not the room has been cleaned without even stepping inside. It has nothing to do with the cleaning process itself. For a long time Michael was understandably annoyed at my seemingly irrational reactions to perfectly nice rooms. Now we know what to do. He is happy to call ahead and request fragrance-free rooms when possible or when we are on a road trip he goes in ahead of me to check the status of monsters in the room. On the other hand, I have always loved the atmosphere surrounding warm indoor hotel swimming pools. The chlorine smell signals a mold-free environment and I am at my happiest when there is no mold to alter my moods.

Sometimes the receipts given out at check-out could cause me to feel upset. After a pleasant hotel experience Michael would enter the car with the freshly printed paperwork in his hand. In just a moment, I would begin to feel uneasy, and frustration ensued because I truly did not know why. Being a man, Michael would want to solve the problem, but there was nothing to solve. It was not about service or facilities. I wasn't nostalgic at the end of vacation. Now we know we can hold that innocent piece of newly-printed paper responsible, and it goes promptly into the trunk, or even better, into the nearest trash bin.

Traveling to Cincinnati to visit family often turned into an allergic nightmare. I would start out excited and happy, looking forward to the trip. As we got closer and closer to the big city, my allergic symptoms began to kick in. By the time we arrived I was tired, coughing, wheezing and unhappy. I tried of course to cover it all up, but the allergens kept piling on. I was never at my best on these occasions and I never knew why, until now.

Of course various industrial pollutants, petrochemicals and vehicles exhausts contributed to increasingly denser air as we approached the city. Road dust has been analyzed to uncover over twenty different possible allergens in addition to those from vehicle exhaust. That was the base. Then a different home environment, including things like house pets, cologne, newspapers and cooking odors as well as different pollens in the air contributed to overwhelming my system. Even if we had understood the power of allergens back then, there was nothing we could do to remove them. I was never a good traveler, no matter how much I loved my family.

Even after I was immunized I was still apprehensive about traveling outside my safe zone. Pollen from such things as coconut palms and Norwegian spruce trees was not typically in my Tennessee serum formula, and there was no way of knowing how I might react to such unknowns. Traveling outside the country is something I can only dream about. We finally discovered that I was allergic to my mother's Tabu perfume. It explained a lot of things, including the fact that I always dreaded and tried to avoid long trips in the car with my parents because I was never at my best in that closed environment. Again, I missed a lot.

We once took Andy's baseball team on a trip to California. For some unknown reason (probably good cabin air filtration) the plane ride presented no problems. The west coast air apparently agreed with me. We stayed in dormitories rather than hotels and I found myself leading the way, riding the subways and trolleys, and walking up and down the hills of San Francisco. It was invigorating, and my energy levels were higher than I could ever remember. It was also a big city, but I reacted in an entirely different way. Even my asthma was not a problem. Not all mysteries have solutions, and I have yet to figure this one out.

When our children were younger, I always hesitated to volunteer for their field trips. Obviously, I couldn't be counted on to drive but I loved to chaperone. I worried that others would assume I just didn't want to volunteer and participate. Of course that was not the case, but my reluctance was hard to explain, and I knew no one would understand, even if I tried. Making up excuses was simply easier. Once again, I missed a lot of memories.

Driving at high speeds along the interstate highways almost always ensured unexpected encounters with road construction, accidents, and other traffic delays. These encounters could mean real trouble. Smelling the tar and asphalt repair fumes could bring on an immediate asthma attack. Slow traffic made things even worse because of the duration of the exposure and my inability to avoid the smelly exhaust fumes. Having to roll the windows down to save fuel from the air conditioner allowed more monsters to invade my space. I was never upset about the unavoidable delays, but nevertheless, my feelings of distress and brain fog were very real. I feel bad for those who have to work in those conditions every day, and I often wonder if these triggers could contribute to frustrated drivers and road rage.

As a driver I never took chances, even though doing so would have come easily had I been so inclined. I was apprehensive about merging onto the interstate, probably because I felt less in control than I actually was, never knowing when "brain fog" might kick in. I know I am not the only one who feels this way, and I have labeled the feeling "emergeaphobia." Michael helps me avoid these situations, mapping things out for me in advance, finding alternate routes when possible and being my second set of eyes.

When our grandchildren were little, one of my favorite responsibilities was taking them places when their parents were at work, and I was the first call number in case of emergency. Of course I always wanted to help, but I panicked whenever the gas tank was less than half full. The mere thought of needing to pump my own gas in an emergency caused me extreme anxiety. If I got sick, I could cause even more of a problem. Michael still keeps the gas tank at least half-full for me, but I always have to know where the closest full-service station is located, just in case.

Vacations were usually less than ideal because even though I didn't want to be, I was high maintenance. Activities such as riding bumper cars with the kids were problematic because of the fumes; the scent of sunscreen on crowded beaches was unavoidable; and going in and out of boutiques, gift shops, and antique stores was a nuisance because of potential allergen-filled air of one sort or another. Someone had to go in first and check things out. Long hours in the sun were impossible for me unless we took along tarps and beach umbrellas. Cedar and natural woods in mountain chalets smell wonderful, but not if you are allergic.

Even floating down a river in a rubber raft or inner tube can be trouble if the hot sun on the rubber causes outgassing. But then I guess falling asleep along the way might not really be so bad. Even the thought of taking a cruise is troubling. I would surely become seasick and then I might be allergic to the anti-nausea medication. If there were perfumes and environmental issues, there would be no escape, and no way to take a "test trip" ahead of time. For now I think I will just keep my feet on dry land. I missed out a lot because of the "maybe's," but I truly hope my clues may help you plan your travel wisely and anticipate possible difficulties ahead of time. Allergies can be managed much more easily when mysteries turn into facts.

I cannot emphasize enough how important my immunizations have been in my life. This past summer we had a wonderful family vacation in the Smoky Mountains. The chalet was beautiful and I smiled the whole time. Floating down the river is amazing and even at my age, zip-lining is my new favorite sport. Life is good!

HIDDEN INGREDIENTS
#pleasedonthideyoursugarinmysalt

Hidden ingredients are an allergic nightmare. These days we all know the importance of reading labels. The process can be confusing and time-consuming, but receiving accurate information is the only way to know what we are putting in our bodies every day. Reading labels from items on supermarket shelves is easy enough, but what we and our families eat when away from home is an entirely different matter. Hidden ingredients are sneaking into our food supply like the legendary Trojan horse. I truly wish these items did not have to be there, but my main concern is the fact that they are not easily recognized so that those of us with food allergy can more clearly identify the items to which we are allergic. If something isn't bad for us, why must it be hidden? In the matter of food allergy, amounts of the allergen are not significant, so secret recipes are not at risk. A reaction can occur whether the offending exposure is a pinch, a spoonful or a cupful. It brings out the detective in me. Jigsaw puzzles are impossible to complete if pieces are missing or distorted.

I began paying attention to labels after my first food allergy test in the 1980s. I was allergic to carrots, and I was shocked to learn that cheese turns orange from adding annatto, a yellow-orange vegetable dye from the achiote tree, carrot juice, chemical dyes like yellow 5 or yellow 3, and even marigold petals. My mother and many other people are allergic to these beautiful summer flowers. Orange cheese is pretty, but it doesn't come from the cow that way. I started preferring naturally white cheese instead, and the flavor is the same. I also avoid cheese slices made from oil and those individually wrapped in plastic which are only required to contain 50% cheese. I am not clear about what comprises the remaining 50%. The mold you find in Roquefort, blue, limburger and brie cheeses is not a problem, unless you are allergic to mold. I once read a story about a lady who broke up with her boyfriend because he thought that Velveeta was real cheese. I guess it pays to be informed.

I am suspicious when I see the words "hypoallergenic" or "allergy friendly" or "produced in an allergy-free facility." These terms are neither medical nor scientific. They are only related to marketing, and there are no government standards involved. The term "hypoallergenic" was invented in 1953 by a cosmetics company developing a new line of makeup. Other companies soon got on the bandwagon. These labels, as well as the phrase "less allergenic" are essentially meaningless because consumers can be allergic to anything. When I see these claims, I ask myself, "Who says?" or "Less than what?" or "How do they know what I am allergic to?" My advice to all of you is simply this: "Buyer Beware."

A tiny bit of any allergen is all that is required to cause a reaction. For example, the small amount of anchovies in a spoonful of Worcestershire sauce or Caesar salad dressing makes them delicious, but be careful if you have a fish allergy.

Processed products can be very complicated. For example, spreadable fruits (as opposed to jams and jellies) can be labeled on the front as "100% fruit." However, the back label tells a different story. The ingredient list on the back of one jar of natural raspberry fruit spread includes fruit syrup, black raspberries, lemon juice concentrate, fruit pectin and natural flavors. My questions are the following: What kind of fruit and what sugars are in the syrup? Are whole lemons used in the concentrate? What fruits are in the pectin? What ingredients are in the "natural flavors?" Maybe you are not allergic to raspberries so you think this is a good single ingredient choice. You could, however, be allergic to pears and strawberries, which could easily be in the syrup. Pectin is a thickening agent, a polysaccharide found in fruits and vegetables. It is generally considered harmless, but it can contain unlisted additives and the fruit of origin is unknown. The insinuation that the product is a single ingredient is misleading.

Full-fat plain yogurt is a very healthy choice. It contains more protein and less sugar than the fat-free versions; but if you are determined to stick with the low fat or fat free products, beware that they most likely contain gelatin, cornstarch, and other additives to attain the creamy texture. Whenever fat is taken out of a food, sugar and salt are frequently added in its place. Live active cultures are often removed in the process as well.

This brings us to the vague term, "natural ingredients." It is a helpful list if you are trying to avoid "unnatural ingredients," but it is not at all helpful if you are trying to identify allergens in your food. The FDA (Food and Drug Administration)[11] refers to natural ingredients as "ingredients extracted directly from plants or animal products as opposed to being produced synthetically." There is no requirement to list the foods from which these ingredients are derived. It could be anything. The list of possibilities is endless.

The ingredient list on most butter boxes reads "cream, salt." In the old days they churned cream until it turned to butter and if desired, they added salt. So it stands to reason that the ingredient list on a box of unsalted butter would simply read, "Cream." Not so. The list reads "cream and natural flavors." Food processors feel the need to replace the salt with unknown ingredients, so instead of a pure product, we have another mystery. It makes no sense to me. I wish I had a butter churn!

Margarine and other processed butter replacement products are regarded by some as a healthy, low-fat alternative. Contrary to the catchy saying, margarine is not really "one molecule away from plastic." It is, however, made of vegetable oil (source often not identified), skim milk, salt, emulsifiers, food additives, and food colorings such as yellow 6, which is derived from petroleum. This coloring has been linked to ADHD and food allergies (as in aspirin) and is banned in many European countries. The term "vegetable oil" generally refers to any plant oil that is liquid at room temperature. Those with allergies to such things as soy, corn and peanuts (not actually nuts) should be aware that these ingredients are often included but not individually identified on labels. Although more expensive and sometimes hard to

---

11 www.fda.gov

find, grass-fed butter is a healthy choice.

If you are allergic to eggs, especially egg whites (albumen), the knowledge that they can pop up in all sorts of unexpected places can be very helpful. I use eggs as an example, but other foods appear unexpectedly as well. Seventy-five billion eggs are produced in the U.S. every year. If you are exposed to any egg protein, your symptoms may develop within minutes of consumption or even several hours later. This is the case with most food allergens, which makes it hard for the consumer to accurately self-diagnose a specific food allergy.

For example, you might have an unknown egg exposure at 10 am (in your coffee, for example) and then at lunch you eat shrimp and a baked potato. Ten minutes after the meal, you break out in hives. You blame the shellfish, when in actuality egg was the culprit. This miscalculation could easily be avoided with an accurate allergy test. How sad to give up shrimp if you don't have to! Eggs appear in a wide range of products such as meatloaf, pretzels, wine (if cleared with egg whites), finger paint, ice cream, laxatives, shampoo, baking powder, pasta, processed meats, marshmallows, root beer, mayonnaise, jelly beans, make-up, sushi and marzipan.

Anyone with an egg allergy should also avoid the flu vaccine, especially the nasal spray version. Labels on nutritional supplements not regulated by the FDA are not required to list "egg" on the ingredient list, but the Mayo Clinic urges anyone allergic to eggs to avoid consuming anything from the following list: albumen, globulin, lecithin, livetin, lysozyme, vitellin, and any words beginning with "ova" or "ovo," such as ovalbumin. They contain eggs.

The term "broth" is not a single ingredient. It is a combination of all sorts of things, unless you make your own. If you come across a three-ingredient recipe which lists the three components as chicken, rice, and chicken broth, don't be fooled. The commercial broth likely contains vegetables, spices, flavor enhancers and preservatives as well as antibiotics, growth hormones and other chemicals found in non-organic beef or chicken products.

If you have a mold allergy, there are certain foods you should try to avoid. Even smelling a food such as milk to see if it is spoiled can set off a reaction from inhaling the mold spores in the air. Once you are immunized, these things are much less of a problem. In the meantime, some foods to avoid are mushrooms, cheese, sour cream, meats which are pickled, cured or smoked, buttermilk, most vinegars, soy sauce, dried fruits, wine, beer, bread and other foods made with yeast. There is even mold in ground black pepper and other dried spices. These foods might not bother you if eaten occasionally, but beware of piling on. In general, I no longer have to worry about these hidden moldy triggers, thanks to Dr. Pienkowski and my allergy shots.

Our forefathers ate wheat, corn, barley and other grains freely, without getting fat. They were unaware of problems with gluten and they baked wonderful breads and cakes which they enjoyed, often several times a day. What went wrong? For one thing, they did not soak their pre-harvest wheat crop with high-octane Roundup weed killer. For the past 15 years, conventional wheat farmers drench their fields with Roundup several days before the harvesters work the fields. Used as a desiccant, it supposedly encourages an easier, earlier, and bigger yield. I know someone who is a commercial wheat farmer. Neighbors come and beg for some of his commercial Roundup which is so much more powerful than the product commonly available for fighting weeds in their gardens and yards.

Glyphosate, the primary ingredient in Roundup, is not considered fatally toxic or poisonous by our government. This does not mean it is safe to eat on a daily basis. It is too soon to determine the long-term effects on our population. This hidden ingredient surely must be a significant problem for those of us with allergies and chemical sensitivities. Organic wheat flour is almost impossible to find in grocery stores. America's wheat and possibly other grain crops such as barley and rye are possibly affected for the next several years, and maybe even forever. We are trapped, because as consumers we have no way of knowing whether or not a product we purchase has been treated with Roundup or any other weed killer. As consumers, we have little way of growing our own wheat, and certainly no way of milling it

into flour. I often wonder if glyphosate is more of a problem than gluten, which has been around for centuries. Scientists are studying the
chemical's relationship to cancer. It is too soon to identify the long-
term effects of genetically modified food products, but I avoid them
whenever I can. Someone has said that what you don't know won't
hurt you. I beg to disagree.

Gluten first appeared during the sixth century as an ingredient for
making Chinese noodles. According to Wikipedia, gluten is the main
protein of wheat. It is made by washing wheat flour dough with water
until all the starch granules have been removed, leaving the sticky insol-
uble gluten as an elastic mass which is then cooled before being eaten.

The terms "wheat" and "gluten" are often used interchangeably,
but they are not the same thing. In recent years, the term "gluten" has
become a buzzword, an ingredient to be strictly avoided as part of
clean healthy eating. "Gluten free" appears on product labels even
when the product could never have included gluten in the first place.
It is the "sticky protein" which helps foods maintain their shape, and
it acts as the glue which binds foods together. It hides in most processed, boxed, and packaged foods such as condiments, deli meats,
canned soups, granola bars, soft drinks and anything which contains
"caramel color." Body care products and cosmetics can also contain
wheat gluten, which can be absorbed through the skin, producing the
same symptoms as if you had eaten it.

Those with celiac disease (a true gluten allergy) and gluten sensitivity experience symptoms such as headache, fatigue, skin rash,
muscle cramps, and digestive issues. This disease is hard to diagnose,
and as many as 80 percent of people with celiac disease are unaware
of their condition. As many as 18 million Americans have a non-
celiac gluten sensitivity.[12]

Since human beings have been eating wheat and its gluten for at
least 10,000 years, I wonder if these health issues have always been
part of our medical history. It makes sense to me that perhaps glyphosate, pesticides, and other man-made artificial ingredients which are

---

12   www.beyondceliac.org

working their way into our wheat products should be studied as contributing factors to these gluten-related issues.

Trace amounts of Roundup and other chemicals are beginning to show up in our organic wheat and other products as well. Their origin is a mystery which is nowhere close to being solved. I wonder if anyone is really even trying.

When I recognized my problem with color-coated tablets and capsules, I soon realized that the medicine itself was most likely not the problem. More likely, the culprit came from within the following list of inactive ingredients associated with products such as Nuprin or Motrin: Carnauba wax, cornstarch, FD&C yellow No. 6, hydroxypropyl methylcellulose, talc, sesame oil, propylene glycol, silicon dioxide, stearic acid, titanium dioxide, acacia, pregelatinized starch, calcium sulfate, povidone, stearic acid, croscarmellose sodium, white wax, sucrose (sugar), and shellac. I have no idea which of these added ingredients cause my allergic reactions so I just try to avoid them all except when absolutely necessary.

If you have problems with additives in your medication, your local compounding center can help by personalizing your prescriptions and eliminating unnecessary ingredients and those to which you are allergic. These amazing pharmacists prepare your medicine the way they did it in the old days, before we gave way to mass producing and mass marketing everything. They can even sometimes help with products other than medicine, such as shampoo and toothpaste. The old is forever new.

If you have an underarm rash, the logical offender would be the deodorant or antiperspirant you use every day, or the shaving cream if you shave under your arms. However, it could also be the formaldehyde present in permanent press clothing. Many people are allergic to formaldehyde. It was declared the Contact Allergen of the Year for 2015 by the American Contact Dermatitis Society (ACDS). It is a volatile organic compound found in both indoor and outdoor air and in numerous products we use every day such as toothpaste, baby wipes, nail polish and paper towels. The Department of Health and Human

Services lists it as a known carcinogen.

To those who are sensitive, these monsters are everywhere. High concentrations of formaldehyde in the home can lead to symptoms such as asthma, rashes, brain fog and fatigue even if you are not chemically allergic. It is more easily released into the air in hot and humid places. Keeping the air as cool as possible is a good idea. You should wash any new clothing and bed linens before using them since manufacturers in the U.S. and some other countries are not required to disclose the inclusion of formaldehyde on their labels. One hundred percent cotton products are often the best choice.

Bed linens made from bamboo are becoming very popular. They are practically wrinkle-free, very soft, and very expensive. After sleeping on a set for several nights, I realized that I was waking up in the mornings with less than usual energy accompanied by feelings of uneasiness and apprehension. I took my own advice and analyzed my sleeping partners. Bamboo sheets were the only new additions. I switched back to my usual linens and the next morning I was back to normal. I experienced no sneezes, no sniffles, and no rash which would have instantly alerted me to an allergy. Nevertheless, something was not right. It did not take long for this sleuth to determine that bamboo is not my friend!

Formaldehyde also appears in cigarette smoke and E-cigarettes. It is even added to processed foods like milk and noodles to increase their shelf life. Formaldehyde inhalants are a key component in that familiar "new car smell" in recently purchased vehicles. Individually, formaldehyde amounts can be minor, but we need to understand how they affect our personal environment. As always, piling on is a large concern and formaldehyde allergy is a serious condition for lots of people. Formaldehyde can be listed by other names such as formalin, methanal, methylene glycol, formic aldehyde, and others.

Sometimes the need for technical knowledge is overwhelming for the general population. The ability to identify these intruders is of paramount importance in any attempt to reduce our exposure. Both forcing these allergens out of hiding and strengthening our defenses against them are worthy goals for all Americans. Our health as a nation depends upon it.

I used to think white vinegar was the best choice for cooking. It looks clean, clear and healthy. I have changed my mind. Research alerted me to the fact that white vinegar is made from corn which is distilled into corn alcohol (moonshine?) then mixed with water and fermented into vinegar. Not a good selection, especially for those with corn allergy, but excellent for household cleaning. My choice is raw apple cider vinegar. It is organic, uncooked, and unfiltered. It also includes "the mother," a complex structure of beneficial acids which are considered very healthy for humans. Of course, if you have apple allergy, this might not be the best vinegar choice for you.

Many people believe that frosting is something spreadable that comes unrefrigerated in a can or plastic tub. I copied the following list of ingredients from a can of vanilla frosting.

The label reads, "Sugar, palm oil, water, corn syrup, cornstarch, canola oil, salt, mono and diglycerides, artificial flavor, artificial color including yellow 5 and red 40, modified cornstarch, polysorbate 60, potassium sorbate, soy lecithin, xanthan gum, citric acid, antioxidants, ascorbyl palmitate, mixed tocopherols, chamomile and rosemary extracts."

Large letters also pronounce it gluten free. Who would put wheat gluten in their frosting in the first place? I wonder why it takes yellow 5 and red 40 to make the icing pure white. And where is the vanilla?

The simple truth is that you can just turn on your hand mixer, whip up some powdered sugar, milk, butter, and a few grains of salt to make the most delicious buttercream frosting you could ever imagine. Add a little cocoa, vanilla flavoring or lemon juice and voila! Perfect frosting with no hidden ingredients. "Maybe next time I will go out to my herb garden and add some chamomile or rosemary to make my frosting taste even better," said this author, NEVER!

It is the same thing with cake mix. A long list of unpronounceable synthetic ingredients appears with flour and sugar on the ingredient label. You still have to mix these dry ingredients together with your own eggs and oil. If you bake from scratch, you only need flour, sugar, shortening, baking powder, milk and salt to bake a delicious cake, the way they used to cook before we all got fat.

Contrary to popular opinion, pure whipped cream does not come in a plastic tub or an aerosol can. Both are full of additives and chemicals. The ingredient list will probably surprise you, but spraying the creamy white foam is still a lot of fun! If you want something really scrumptious, open a carton of pure whipping cream. Turn on the beaters and sprinkle in a little sugar. The result is amazingly delicious.

Sometimes a hidden ingredient is actually an organism inside the food itself. If you experience an allergic reaction after a fish dinner, the offender might not be the fish. It could be a parasite called anisakis, commonly located in temperate waters around the world. It can affect fish and squid and has even been found to cause reactions from casual contact by factory workers. Possible reactions include asthma, hives, digestive trauma and anaphylaxis. I only mention this to point out that food allergy tests identify specific troublesome foods and can also serve to eliminate contributing factors in certain medical emergencies. If the patient is not allergic to fish, other culprits such as the parasite would have to be considered. Cold water fish, such as wild-caught Alaskan salmon, are not affected.

Other hidden ingredients I have come across through the years include such things as sugar added to salt and stevia powder, peanut butter in sauces, wood cellulose and mold inhibitors in grated cheese, red food dye in farm-raised salmon, shrimp, and other shellfish, rice in Michelob beer and canned biscuits, sugar in lipstick, calcium chloride and citric acid in canned tomatoes and other vegetables, and a mysterious "15% solution" in packaged meats.

I once asked the meat manager in one of the major food chains if she could tell me what was in the solution which was injected into their meat products such as pork chops, steak, and chicken. She was clueless and referred me to the general manager. He had no idea, and called home office. No one knew, or if they did they would not say. I asked if he could help me find a product that was "just meat." He could not. I changed stores.

Enhanced meat is becoming more and more popular in our country today. As I understand it, fresh meat is passed through a computerized machine which pierces it with tiny needles, injecting it with water and various other ingredients such as salt, phosphates, antioxidants and flavorings. This unidentified solution can extend the shelf life of the meat by 30 to 50 percent.

In the matter of pork for example, meat processing facilities are replacing the natural fat (and flavor) which has been intentionally bred out of the animal in an attempt to make it more appealing to health-conscious consumers. This process, also called "plumping," makes no sense to me, as it seems that natural ingredients are being exchanged for artificial ones. There must also be a cost factor involved in putting something back in that you previously took out. Even seasonings such as teriyaki sauce can be injected into the meat.

Arsenic in "acceptable amounts" is sometimes added to chicken feed to prevent parasitic infection and make the meat look fresh and pink. Its use was regulated in America in 2013, but details of all these unnatural additives are not readily available to the public.

The term "all natural" on the label does not guarantee unenhanced meat. If you shop in the unpackaged meat section and the clerk says their meat is not enhanced, ask to see the original box or the Cryovac packaging because chances are they do not really know for sure. As consumers, we need to know what we are eating. Even though someone else decides which ingredients pass as healthy, those of us with food allergy have a special need to know what personal allergens might be hiding in the foods we eat. What is healthy for one person could be fatal for someone else.

If you have never tasted homemade mayonnaise, you are missing a real treat. I remember watching my grandmother make it. She insisted it was the only thing you could eat on a tomato sandwich. She had the patience of Job as she whipped it up, adding half a cup of Wesson oil, drop by drop to get the emulsion just right. Today there are lots of unnecessary ingredients in store-bought mayonnaise. If you have a stick blender and a wide-mouth jar, you can make your own. Simply pour in one eight-ounce bottle of light olive oil, one large egg and one yolk, one tablespoon of fresh lemon juice, a large pinch of dry mustard, a few grains of sugar or stevia, and a large pinch of salt. Blend for a few seconds and watch as it magically emulsifies into creamy mayonnaise. With a little experimenting with the amounts of the seasonings to suit your taste, you will soon produce a product even better than Hellman's or Duke's.

Shredding a block of cheese only takes a couple of minutes, especially if you have a food processor. It is much more delicious than processed grated cheese in a bag, and with no added products from the wood-chipper! Mix your mayonnaise and cheese, add a jar of pimentos, and you will have an easy, delicious batch of pure home-made Carolina Cavar (better known as pimento cheese).

Food shopping can be very confusing for anyone with a milk allergy. Products labeled "non-dairy" may still contain milk-derived ingredients such as casein, curd, hydrolysates, lactose, rennet, and whey. Lactose intolerance is often confused with milk allergy, but even though they are both problematic, they are not the same thing. Lactose intolerance occurs when the body can't digest lactose, the sugar found in dairy products. Ingestion produces stomach pain, diarrhea, and gas. Milk allergy means that your immune system identifies the dairy exposure as a foreign agent and goes after it by releasing histamines. Symptoms can be wheezing, vomiting, headache, rash, and so forth. If you are allergic to cow's milk, many alternatives are available, such as soy milk, rice milk, goat milk, coconut milk, and almond milk. Some have added ingredients, but sampling them is worth a try if you are sensitive to dairy products.

Buying shredded wheat or another type of cereal to avoid corn is a good idea if you are allergic, but you should know that cornstarch is often used to powder the inside of the bags. It is a hidden ingredient because the cereal itself is corn-free, and the starch doesn't have to be listed. I don't know how we know if the cornstarch is there or not. I have never seen it. Another mystery.

I don't know how you feel about cooking sprays in aerosol cans. I prefer brushing on a thin layer of melted butter or olive oil with a basting brush. There are also inexpensive oil misters which you fill with your own preferred cooking oil. I like to avoid all the chemicals and propellants whenever possible, but there is another reason to be cautious with these products and read the labels carefully. Most of them contain soy derivatives, rosemary extract and other possible unexpected food allergens. They can be easily inhaled and absorbed by the foods we eat.

Fast food, take-out and home-delivery are conveniences impossible to avoid these days. Many of us are drawn like giant magnets to drive-through windows and pizza parlors. We love our cocktails, restaurant meals and movie theater popcorn. We order pre-made boxed meals in attempts to lose weight or we grab a boxed dinner from the grocer's freezer. I am not suggesting we have to give up these occasional choices, but we do need to be aware of what we are eating, including those hidden ingredients no one likes to think about. Ingredient awareness is crucial in any attempt to do a better job of rotating foods and avoiding the piling on factor whenever food allergy is involved.

When eating away from home, we need to know what questions to ask, especially if the allergy is severe. I like to know if my potatoes are mashed in the kitchen or re-created with dehydrated flakes from a cardboard box. In times past, restaurant meals were a special treat and people didn't have to worry about hidden ingredients, but times have changed. Salad bars are sprayed with preservatives, and grill marks are often just some dark-colored solution stamped or painted on with a brush. Many times the restaurants don't even know what is in the products they use. I don't know why it is such a secret, but reluctance to divulge ingredients makes me suspicious.

Every Christmas when we unpack our 40-year collection of mostly handmade tree ornaments, a special yet simple one always catches my eye. One year my Montessori preschoolers made ornaments by stringing colorful Fruit Loops cereal onto narrow ribbon, then tying them into a circle to hang on the tree branch. Many children had just learned how to tie a bow, and they were especially proud to show off their newly acquired skills. That was in 1990.

Even with no special handling, not a single one of those tiny loops of cereal has ever faded, crumbled, or broken. I mention this to illustrate the power of preservatives in our food supply. It raises many questions such as, "How long will these preservatives stay in our bodies? What effect do these additives have on our systems? Do our bodies ever really get rid of these chemicals or will they preserve us into antiquity? Will they eventually petrify our organs? I am indulging in a bit of absurdity of course, but it does make you wonder, and only time will tell.

If all of this seems overwhelming to you, I hope you will resist the urge to just give up. Most people are not as allergic as I am, and maybe you only need to avoid one or two foods. If you are not chemically sensitive, these hidden additives will probably not cause problems if eaten in moderation. Being more informed helps us all to make better choices. For a long time I did not make the connection between unknown symptoms and food allergy. Now I know that the day after a special occasion I may not feel my best, but at least I know why, and it is worth it. As my detective work continues and more and more ingredients come out of hiding, I am much less allergified. I am pretty sure you will be too.

Most of all, we should be able to take the time to enjoy our food. We can be diligent while never letting the latest discoveries and opinions create a constant concern. Food choices should not become an everyday annoyance; that in itself would be unhealthy. As George Bernard Shaw once said, "There is no love sincerer than the love of food."

When Monsters Attack Body Parts
BACKACHE
#ohmyachingbackatleastitsjustthefoodandnottherheumatiz

Back problems have been a major source of extreme pain and discomfort for too many Americans for too many years. I have read that at least 80 percent of the population experience some form of lower back pain at some time in their lives.[13] It is the second most common cause of disability and is responsible for untold hours of missed work every year. Often the problem can be identified and corrected, but sometimes it is illusive and pain management is the only answer. Chronic backache is held consistently responsible for untold opioid addictions which have plagued our modern society for decades.

I have had persistent and intractable back pain and muscle spasms throughout my life. As a result of my victory over the monsters, I no longer have any back problems or discomfort whatsoever. The cure has nothing to do with pain pills, exercise, acupuncture or surgery. Allergy was the problem all along.

Beginning in my mid-twenties, pain in my lower back region was intermittent and non-specific. Often by the time I felt like going to the doctor, the pain would diminish. I learned to deal with it. It could be severe, but never lasted more than a week or so. Then it would return without warning in various stages of intensity. From time to time I was diagnosed with such things as skeletal muscle strain, pulled muscles in the back area, sciatica, and arthritis. None of it made sense to me. How could a skeletal muscle strain clear up in three to four days? I was once told it was a kidney problem, probably stones, and I should watch my calcium intake. "Perhaps it is a sponge kidney," my doctor said, and changed the subject. Nothing ever came of that diagnosis, and as far as I know, both my kidneys are perfectly fine and I have never passed a kidney stone.

While working in our flower shop, I would often have a sore back and from time to time sharp pain would shoot down from my hips to my ankles. It mimicked sciatica, but when the doctors ruled that condition out, the pains persisted. The only advice I ever received was that I was on my feet too long, standing at my work station on the hard cement and I should find a mat or piece of carpeting to cushion the floor. I should also experiment with different types of shoes. This

---

13   www.acatoday.org

advice made no sense to me because other staff and designers were in the same category and they never complained of any back discomfort. Thankfully it wasn't constant, but back pain definitely interfered with my quality of life.

Once when I was getting a pedicure, I had an extremely severe back spasm and I could not get out of the chair. I couldn't move. Everyone wanted to call 911, but I convinced them to wait for a while. Eventually the pain subsided, and everything was back to normal with no residual pain. It happened several times, but no cause was ever found. Sometimes it felt like a giant bubble, rolling around inside my body and pressing against my spine.

As a Montessori teacher, I had to move furniture, carry young children, and sit cross-legged with them on the floor. As my back problems became more prevalent, I was afraid I was going to have to give up my job. My family doctor reluctantly ordered x-rays. We looked at the results together and he said, pointing to an obviously swollen area in my lower back, "As you can see, that is clearly arthritis." I wasn't really sure what I was seeing, but he was the doctor and I took his word for it. "Your only hope," he continued, "is to exercise. It will never go away." I was devastated, but not convinced.

By the time I got to Dr. Pienkowski, I was afraid I had a tumor. He soothed my fears and explained that the swelling in my back was caused by allergy, and it would go away with treatment. He was right.

I see television infomercials, magazine articles, advice columns, commercials, talk shows, and news broadcasts, all offering various products and services guaranteed to provide relief from aching backs. Ergonomic office equipment, mattresses, pillows, heating pads, creams, exercise machines, orthotic shoe inserts, medications, surgery and pain management clinics are advertised to provide the perfect pain-free solution. Never once have I heard the word allergy mentioned in these articles. References to food allergy as a contributing factor to back pain rarely appear in all of my research online, but more and more positive studies are being conducted. If you have a swollen abdomen (possibly allergy-related), your skeletal system is likely out of joint and the risk of back injury from bending and lifting is much more prevalent.

In the 1920s Dr. S. H. Rowe discovered that chronic muscular pain often had a food allergy connection and in the 1950s Dr. A. H. Rinkel listed low back pain as one of the symptoms of allergy. I guess no one was interested enough to take them seriously. In 1989 Dr. Marek Pienkowski determined that my back pain was caused by allergy, particularly food allergy, and he was correct. Subsequent studies have further verified the connection.

The term "allergic cascade" is the medical term used to describe a sequence of chemical releases that takes place in response to the body's exposure to allergens. Sue Killian of the Institute for Therapeutic Discovery and John McMichael of Beech Tree Laboratories recently conducted several studies on the allergy connection to back pain and they concluded that, "While obvious injuries are readily diagnosed, finding and treating non-specific back pain is more challenging. Investigating the connection between allergy and back pain reveals that the allergic cascade produces some of the same inflammatory cytokines and neuropeptides which produce back pain. If allergies are concurrent with back pain, treating the allergies often has a positive effect because controlling the allergic cascade diminishes the addition of chemicals common to both conditions."[14] This information is very encouraging and should definitely be considered as a possible answer for anyone who suffers from unidentified back pain which does not respond to traditional treatments.

Dr. Pienkowski eliminated my back problems with his precise diagnosis and immunotherapy treatment. For that I am forever grateful. Hopefully allergy will soon become more generally recognized and accepted as a possible contributing factor to the mystery of illusive back pain. If you are looking for the missing pieces to your own seemingly unsolvable backache puzzle, perhaps you will find them here.

____

14 Journal of Allergy Disorders and Therapy, Vol. 2, Issue 1, 2015, 1-4

COUGHING
#popcornearthquakesconcertsandcandy

I was raised in a large southern family which appreciated the importance of decorum, good manners and the social graces. One did not create a spectacle in public places. One did not talk loudly and disturb others in restaurants or theaters, and especially not in church. It was a matter of respect. When my allergic coughing spasms were such an issue, it was easier for me to just stay home, collapsed in a heap under the covers, recovering from the day before. I feared that those around me would think I was contagious and spreading some terrible disease. I would never be that insensitive, and since I coughed so much of the time, I missed a lot but my faith never faltered. I wonder what my previous generations of ancestors would think about my current crusade to find a cure for chronic coughing. I hope they would be proud.

Even at home I tried my hardest not to disturb Michael and the children. They always reassured me and said it didn't matter, but it mattered to me. Extreme episodes were becoming more frequent in the 1980s, and I would cough so hard the muscles in my chest and abdomen would ache for days. Still the doctors continued to treat my symptoms, which always came back, often with a vengeance.

My normally soft voice could suddenly erupt like the roar of a lion and the pattern continued. I was a non-smoker and was never diagnosed with any disease other than those associated with my asthma and allergies. I always had a tickle, or an itchy throat, or a wheezy chest, or what felt like a river running down the back of my throat. It might have been a seasonal situation, but all the seasons ran together and overlapped so that breaks in between were barely noticeable. I know it seems impossible, but coughing just became part of my life. Once I found Dr. Pienkowski, I could rule out cancer or some other horrible dreaded disease, but coughing altered my life and affected me and those around me for years in ways that I am just now beginning to understand.

There were so many different coughs that we decided to give

them each a name. It was the family's attempt to help me deal with the condition on a lighter note, and I love them for all their efforts. The loudest was the Earthquake Cough. It shook our world. It came on usually late at night and sounded as if I were coughing into a bullhorn. I don't know how Michael got any sleep at all, but he seldom left my side. The children eventually learned not to worry and to go back to sleep if it woke them up, but late one night when Andy was about 10 years old, he came rushing into our bedroom, breathlessly yelling, "What's wrong, is it an earthquake?" From then on, we named it the Earthquake Cough, and it continued to shake the house at least twice every year with my predictable bouts of bronchitis every spring and every fall.

I could get some relief with the super-strong cough suppressants prescribed by my family doctor. They were effective for a while, but seldom lasted throughout the night. The few calm hours provided welcome relief from all the stressful and depressing symptoms which accompanied these coughing episodes, but addiction was not an acceptable alternative, and I knew there had to be a better answer. I wanted my health back, and I knew I had to have a clear head if I were ever going to figure it all out. No one else knew what to do. The detective work was all up to me.

Less violent, quieter coughing episodes became known as the Popcorn Cough. These coughs were constant and annoying but not so loud. They were with me all throughout the day, unless I was eating. And I did love to eat! Michael came up with the idea of Movie Popcorn. He would take me to a long movie, usually a matinee because there were fewer people in the theater, and purchase a large bucket of buttery popped corn. Being self-employed, he could arrange his schedule around my coughing episodes, which was a blessing. I learned to eat the popcorn kernel by kernel, and I learned to make it last throughout the entire film. I don't remember many of the movies because I was mostly concentrating on suppressing the cough, but it is a good example of making the best of a difficult situation! Today I hardly cough at all thanks to my successful allergy treatments, but whenever I want to suggest an evening out at the movies, I just tell Michael I have a Popcorn Cough, and he is happy to oblige.

Every spring, fall, and Christmas when Jennifer was in junior high school, she sang in the choral concerts. No matter my current health status, I was determined not to miss any of her performances. They were big productions and were professionally recorded on cassette tape. I was always in the audience, with my own personal coughing concert accompanying me. Medicine helped me manage, but there is proof that I was there. My familiar coughing is clearly in the background on every single tape. The Concert Cough is famous!

The Choker was the most embarrassing cough of all. I would cough so hard I would gag, and it was awful. This condition really affected our quality of life. I refused to go out in public, and I really just wanted to hide in my bedroom to keep the family from having to experience it as well. It was so indelicate and I was so out of control. During these spells, any social life at all was impossible. I felt helpless at times but one thing was certain. The Choker was not going to win.

Getting a good night's sleep is always difficult for those who have coughing problems. I remember as a young child, my mother and I would spend many nights together, propped up in bed, back to back, trying to sleep. Whenever we dozed off, I would slide down to my pillow, and the coughing spasms would wake us up again. The cycle continued. We knew it was asthma, but no one had a good solution. Again, cough medicine worked for a few hours but never lasted through the night. Most of it tasted like bitter licorice, but the "new and improved" cherry-flavored syrupy red #5 stuff was even worse. I hated it.

As an adult I often tried to soothe the hacking cough by falling asleep sucking on a hard peppermint candy or a sugary cough drop. During the coughing seasons there was always a handy candy dish on the bedside table. By God's Grace, I didn't choke to death in my sleep and I do not recommend this solution to anyone. I am also amazed by the fact that after all the many hours they spent bathed in sugar, my teeth didn't fall out! The Candy Cough was anything but sweet.

After I met Dr. Pienkowski, the coughing episodes gradually diminished. Small white uncoated guaifenesin tablets replaced the strong codeine and sugary artificially colored and flavored syrups. Inhalers, particularly rescue inhalers helped me manage sudden coughing attacks, and I was beginning to gain control. As the allergy connection became clear, the fear of unknown scary causes such as lung cancer, heart disease, blood disorders, pleurisy and pneumonia faded away.

Now that my allergies and their constant congestion are in remission, I rarely cough at all and I sleep soundly for eight hours every night. I love being out in public without any fear of embarrassment or sudden attacks. Even public speaking is a joy. In my case, allergy is the only cough explanation ever uncovered, and its far-reaching effects, not only on my health but also on my social life, are thankfully buried in the past. That being said, I vow never to give up my crusade to find a cure for chronic coughing. It is a worthy endeavor.

RESTLESS LEGS
#nervoustwitchyachyfroglegs

Restless Legs Syndrome (RLS) is characterized as a sleep disorder. It is thought to be caused by a change in brain chemistry causing neurons (brain cells) to misfire, creating confusion and disorder in the central nervous system. Twelve million Americans, roughly ten percent of the population, complain of restless legs. Clinics, creams, medications and supplements are widely advertised as help in relieving the severity of restless legs syndrome, but there is no cure. It is often overlooked and misdiagnosed. I have found very little mention of allergy as a contributing factor. In my personal experience, food allergy plays a part.

I have always had restless legs. It usually happens in bed at night when I am trying to get to sleep. However, my restless legs also choose to make an appearance at times other than when I am trying to sleep. The condition really isn't painful, just an aggravating twitching and jumping, sometimes accompanied by an uneasy achy feeling. This annoying involuntary leg movement keeps both of us awake, sometimes off and on for several hours. At other times, it only lasts a few minutes. I have often wondered why it doesn't affect my arms or other parts of my body, but it is always just my legs. Like a frog, jumping off a lily pad, over and over and over again.

Sometimes it begins earlier in the evening after dinner while I am sitting in my comfortable chair, reading my Kindle or watching television. I keep changing positions, and then I can't sit still. The feelings escalate to an uncontrollable urge to move my legs. It is like small muscle spasms but not painful as in cramps. It doesn't always happen at night. Sometimes it happens when we travel and I am sitting in the car for an extended period of time. My legs just won't stay still. I have learned that running while sitting will get you nowhere.

By journaling the dates, times and frequency, along with accompanying circumstances, I was able to make the connection to food. At night, my reactions usually appear an hour or so after dinner. In the car it is usually after we stop for food. Long John Silvers was the first specific observation I made and it was the most consistent. In 2004, I observed a connection between egg whites, sour cream, white rice, mayonnaise, buttermilk ice cream, white flour and cottage cheese. These ingredients are prevalent in such things as fish batter, coleslaw, hushpuppies, and tartar sauce. Not so prevalent in hamburgers and French fries. These ingredients appear less often at breakfast or lunch, which makes sense of the fact that most of my reactions occur in the evening. Strangely enough, there seems to be a connection with the color white.

Of course I can't say that these white foods cause restless legs syndrome. That would be ridiculous. However, I can say that when my legs become restless and I think back to what I have most recently eaten, a version of at least one and often more of these foods were on the menu. To me, this is a definite food allergy connection. I love to eat at Long John Silvers. Now I manage it by eating earlier in the day or making sure I can walk around for a while after the meal. I make other choices if my legs will be trapped in the front seat while travelling in the car. Because I am immunized and not piling on as before, my episodes have become mild and occasional. The intensity is less severe and a couple of aspirin tablets relax my leg muscles so I can drift right off to sleep. These days, I seldom hear Michael say "Oh, your legs are jumping." He doesn't even notice anymore.

Now that I have a better understanding of what is going on, managing my symptoms is much easier. For example, if I know we are going to a wedding and I will have to sit still in church for a long time, I am extra careful about what I eat ahead of time. Then I can splurge on the white cake and fancy foods at the reception, and dance! Sometimes I just eat what I want, knowing that if my legs are twitching I will deal with it. I can get up, take aspirin and walk around a bit. It is less of a problem if I know I don't have to get up early the next morning. Sometimes the foods don't bother me at all, but so far I haven't learned how to predict the outcome. I smile when I see advertisements for restless leg creams which promise to "help calm and soothe those annoying occurrences." If only it were that simple.

There may be a gene connection with restless legs. According to what I read online, over half of the patients treated for restless leg syndrome report at least one family member with a similar condition. This is also true with allergies. My father suffered with restless legs for years. His only medical advice was to exercise. It never really helped him at all.

For certain individuals, various allergy medications, including sedating antihistamines may even worsen the condition. If so, this explains why my restless legs were more bothersome when I was on all the allergy medications and less so after I was immunized. A good night's sleep is just one more reason to be thankful for Dr. Pienkowski.

Hands and Feet
#palmsandsolesandtipsandtoes

Cracked heels and paper thin finger nails plagued me for years. Occasional episodes of athlete's foot, swollen knuckles, tingling fingers and numbness in the fingertips have also been present from time to time. The things we just deal with as minor nuisances increase as the pain reaches a certain level. One at a time, it is not so bad, but when they all flare up at once, it becomes a different story.

In 1998, I began an artistic mosaic tile wall project in our kitchen. I ended up using my fingers to apply the grout between the irregular tiles which I created by wrapping collected china pieces in a towel and smashing them with a hammer. Plastic gloves would have been a wise choice, but they got in my way and were quickly discarded. Soon thereafter my nails became splotchy and sore. I noticed what appeared to be some sort of discoloration, mainly under the tips of my nails. I suspected a nail fungus.

I began going to a nail salon for the first time, and the technicians helped me with manicures and anti-fungal drops, but the condition would not go away. My toenails remained healthy and strong. Our family doctor had no solution for the problem other than to avoid polish, keep my nails short and my hands clean. These tasks were easily accomplished because my nails refused to grow long anyway, no matter how hard I tried. I believe I must have been allergic to the grout.

A friend suggested that I consider having acrylic coatings applied to my nails, which was a fairly new concept at the time. My doctor was skeptical, insisting that I remove the acrylics on a regular basis, to let them breathe. I diligently medicated the nails until they were reasonably clear, and then I had the acrylics professionally applied. Fortunately for me, I was not allergic to the acrylic solution and the process was successful. The hard protective coating provides a barrier which protects the natural nails from absorbing all the harsh chemical products to which our hands are exposed on a daily basis.

Ever since that revelation I have had no more fingernail problems. Underneath the acrylic protective coating, my natural nails are healthy and strong. Some people consider acrylic nails to be a purely cosmetic procedure. To me it is a medical issue that has become a necessity for healthy hands. Of course, if you are allergic to acrylic, this coating is not the answer for you but there are others gels and powders available in salons. Another helpful hint when working with substances such as garden soil is to put a layer of coconut oil under your fingernail tips. Vaseline used to be suggested, but coconut oil is even better because it is anti-fungal. The object is to protect the skin and the nails from possible allergens whenever possible.

Swollen knuckles are not always painful, but they are an indicator of my general state of allergification. When my wedding rings get tight, soap becomes trapped underneath the bands and my skin around them becomes itchy and red. Sometimes my costume jewelry refuses to slide onto my fingers or my toes. It alerts me to the fact that I need to pay attention to what is going on in my system, especially where food allergy is concerned. Michael does what he calls "the finger test" to determine if he is experiencing allergy-related swelling. He laces the fingers of his hands together and then pulls them gently apart. If there is resistance, he knows to keep a better eye on the foods he is eating. It works well, alerting him to a possible allergen overload.

Back in the early days when we were busy with the florist business, my fingertips would sometimes become numb, and there was a tingling sensation in my hands. At times I could lose feeling in them altogether. This was scary when I was the main designer and many people were counting on me for weddings, funerals, anniversaries, and other special occasions with their related deadlines. Back then there were no fresh flowers in grocery stores and you obviously couldn't order online. Floral shops were the only available source and flowers played a much larger role in people's daily lives than they do now. Our delivery trucks were on the road non-stop, all day long. There were very few local businesses which didn't display at least one of our bouquets on someone's desk. An unbelievable amount of pressure accompanied the pleasure we provided. Keeping up with all the orders would have been a challenge even if I hadn't been allergified. It saddens me that people are missing out on the beautiful artistic arrangements which decorated our lives in the past. Artistry back then required so much more than simply jamming a handful of flowers into a plain glass vase. I miss it still, but I digress. . .

My doctor ran tests in an effort to identify the cause of numbness in my hands. He could find no physical disability other than the fact that I have a form of genetic Carpal Tunnel Syndrome which causes occasional compression on the median nerve. He tried to convince me that this was the cause of my "discomfort" and that I was exaggerating my complaints. "Decrease your work load," he said, "and it will go away." This advice was impossible. We had a business to run and I wanted it to be perfect. I was apprehensive because seemingly that sort of physical complaint could quickly turn into a chronic condition, especially since I did the same kind of work every day. The pain and numbness remained intermittent and seemed to flare up along with stressful situations. Once again, I had to be my own detective. I believe I was experiencing a form of panic attack. Too many things, mostly allergy-related, were out of my control. My overloaded immune system was sending me a message that too many conditions were contributing a negative impact on my body. I needed help, but had no idea where to find it. Allergy does indeed affect behavior, both physical and mental.

One time in the early 2000s, Michael was experiencing some trouble with his feet. A dry white rash around the heels and sides along with some nail discoloration indicated athlete's foot. The family doctor prescribed Econazole cream. Dr. Pienkowski referred him to a podiatrist who changed the prescription to Naftin and Lamisil. These medicines cleared up the condition permanently and the Econazole cream wasn't needed. It remained in the medicine cabinet. Soon after his diagnosis, my toes began to itch, just slightly. Knowing that athlete's foot could be contagious, I decided to use some of the Econazole cream, just in case.

It is always a bad idea to use someone else's medication, even if it is just a seemingly harmless foot cream. Soon after the second application, I developed flu-like symptoms and a rare asthma flare-up. I had taken my flu shot, so I suspected allergy and went to see Dr. P. He asked if I had experienced any unusual exposures. Not suspecting the cream, I said no, none that I was aware of. He thought it might be time for re-testing and prescribed my asthma inhaler, Singulair, and Zyrtec. As I walked out the door I remembered the cream, and went back in to tell the nurse. She rushed down the hall to tell the doctor and he made the connection immediately. He changed my prescriptions to Fluconazole, five tablets on alternate days. This medicine, the same one used for female yeast infections, worked right away. It also helped my throat, which I didn't realize had a slight white coating, also related to fungus. We tore up the other prescriptions, which were no longer needed.

We went ahead with another allergy test. Normally I would wear socks when lying face down for the skin test on my back. This time I was barefoot. Dr. Pienkowski noticed the cracks in my heels for the first time. They were deep and painful but I had never mentioned the condition to him before. He said the cracks were related to food allergy. I had always just assumed they were the result of this Tennessee girl going barefoot all year, indoors and out. I was wrong.

I began taking better care of my feet after that. Like the tongue, feet have a lot to say about the condition of one's health. I read a story about a man whose wife was constantly suffering with chest congestion, coughing and wheezing. She was using Vicks Vapo Rub with limited success, applying it inside her nostrils to help her breathe better. For some reason, she ended up rubbing her feet all over with the soothing ointment. She found relief almost instantly. The man was convinced that his wife absorbed the medicine through her feet and it quickly traveled to her upper body, helping her breathe better.

I have no idea if his experience represents a medically accepted fact, but it raised my consciousness and I began paying much more attention to my feet. In actuality, you can detect everything from nutritional deficiencies to diabetes just by looking at your feet. The two feet together contain one fourth of all the body's bones. Each foot also has 100 tendons, 33 joints, ligaments, muscles, nerves and blood vessels that form a network linking all the way up to the heart, spine, and brain.

I replaced my constantly barefoot condition with clean white socks and washable flip-flops. As my allergies improved, so did my painful cracked heels. I still rub my feet with pure coconut oil every chance I get and my heels remain healthy and crack-free. Pedicures have graduated from dreaded medical necessities to occasional luxuries as sandal season approaches. Happy feet prevail, and they dance!

Teeth

#novocainemayeasethepainbutmercurybringsitbackagain

There is even an allergy connection to my teeth. Unlike my mother who wore dentures her whole adult life because her body did not process calcium correctly, my teeth have always been straight and strong. Like so many in my age group, I had a lot of amalgam fillings, usually consisting of 50 percent mercury along with silver, copper, tin and zinc. Mercury is a powerful neurotoxin and at certain levels can cause autoimmune disease, chronic illnesses, and mental disorders. It has been the most common filling material for the last 150 years. Through the years, most of my mercury fillings have been replaced with composite resin or porcelain. I remember as a child playing with the little balls of "quicksilver" in the palm of my hand while waiting for the dentist to fill my cavity. We now know that these fillings release mercury vapor which can be absorbed into the body. It can pose a serious problem for people with chemical allergies, especially to those few who are specifically allergic to mercury.

I didn't mind the shots of novocaine or the sound of the drill, but like most people, I dreaded visits to the dentist. After the procedure to replace the fillings I always felt nauseated and had to sleep it off for a couple of hours when I got back home. I felt vaguely unwell for a week or so afterwards. I knew something was affecting me, but there was no way to know if it was the novocaine, the flavored mouth wash, the fluoride, or something else entirely. It could even have been the dentist's aftershave or his assistant's cologne. I never suspected mercury.

Most likely I did not inherit this aversion to dentistry from my dad's side of the family, but we shared a novocaine problem. He hated it so much that he convinced Dr. Wilson to eliminate the needle and just let him tough it out. Just thinking about it makes me cringe. Later on, Dr. Wilson told me that my dad was the only person he knew who would stop by his dental office on a Saturday morning, "just to say hello." To me, dental office avoidance was a much better idea.

One dental experience in the 1990s was particularly alarming. I needed a root canal and it required anesthesia. I worried about the whole situation and not knowing the dentist, I didn't know what to expect. The procedure went well. Michael took me home, tucked me into bed and went off to work. Sometime later, I woke up from a deep sleep to the sound of the telephone ringing out in the kitchen. There were no cell phones back then so I had to get out of bed to go answer it. I passed out halfway between the bedroom and the kitchen. I woke up on the floor about three hours later. I remember having a terrible headache, tightness in my chest, and I couldn't quit shivering. I called the dental office right away. The receptionist explained that the dentist had called earlier to check on my condition but when no one answered, he assumed I was okay. "Just take a couple of aspirin tablets," she said. "It is nothing to worry about." I am lucky it was not anaphylaxis. I could be dead.

Needless to say, I didn't use that dentist again. I was frustrated because no one seemed to understand the severity of my reactions. My trips to the dentist were different from those of most people. These reactions remain unsolved mysteries, but I have my suspicions.

On dental visits I refuse the flavored mouthwash in favor of filtered water. I choose the most natural products for my professional cleanings, and thankfully mercury fillings are a thing of the past. When I began avoiding artificial ingredients I realized that even toothpaste was a potential problem. I switched to baking soda for a while but then I discovered coconut oil. I use unflavored flossers, I limit my sugar, and I brush twice a day with baking soda or pure unrefined coconut oil. I haven't had a cavity in years, and my twice yearly cleanings are a pleasant experience. I might even stop by one Saturday morning, just to say hello.

There will be more about mercury vapor later in the book.

Ears

#stoppedupachynoisyearsareoftenallergyinduced

Allergy is often responsible for causing excruciating earache pain. I am amazed at how few people associate allergy with any sort of ear problems. As an allergic young child, I remember hiding behind a door or cringing in a corner, holding my breath, afraid of the agonizing pain I would feel if I had to burp or yawn. My ears were constantly infected (otitis media). This condition occurs when bacteria invade the middle ear, causing it to fill with fluid which is then trapped inside. Intense pain occurs as the fluid build-up increases pressure on the eardrum. My pediatrician once told me me never to put anything smaller than my elbow in my ear. It was good advice, of course, and I followed his instructions, but my ears still got stopped up.

As far as I know, no one made the allergy connection back then, but I am making it now. I recall two treatments which were used to help ease my pain. The first was the application of warm oily eardrops. I would lie on my side while my mother used an eyedropper to apply a few drops into each ear. Sometimes she would hold an ice cube in her hand and let the cold drops trickle into my ear to temporarily numb the pain. Both these techniques were soothing, but I always knew the pain would return. Antibiotics, of course, were frequently prescribed. Eventually my frequent earaches subsided, but whenever I was sick, the fluid would build up again.

Numbing the earache pain is temporarily helpful but does nothing to prevent the problems from returning. Many of us, especially children, encounter multiple ear infections throughout the years. Middle ear infections can cause both permanent hearing problems and speech delays in young children, and ear problems are among the most prevalent health issues faced by pediatricians

Nowadays we have access to much better pain management and lots of children go through surgery to have tubes put into their ears.

This surgical procedure is called myringotomy and it requires anesthesia. A small incision is made in the eardrum. Fluid is suctioned out and a tiny barrel-shaped tube is inserted. This procedure permits the fluid to continually drain from the ear. Fresh air then enters the middle ear, allowing it to dry out. Sometimes the tubes fall out prematurely and the whole procedure has to be repeated. I would much prefer to have a specialist like Dr. Pienkowski figure out how to prevent the fluid build-up in the first place. It can be done.

Michael's sister Penny had a severe ear infection at age nine. It turned into a mastoid infection affecting both the middle and inner ear. The military doctors later admitted that had it been treated sooner and had they administered a shot of penicillin when the problem first presented, that devastating condition and its accompanying brain infection could have been prevented. As a result of something beginning with a simple earache, she now has a metal plate in her brain behind the ear as a result of multiple surgeries. Balance issues prevent her from walking unassisted, her hearing is impaired, and she is permanently blind. Because one cannot sue the military, no compensation was ever awarded to this sweet child and her family.

I have always heard ear noises sounding like crumpling paper, and sometimes as loud as radio static. The cacophony is not painful but very annoying. Often when I swallow, I hear loud crackling noises or the muffled sounds of a drum being hit with a rubber mallet. The condition is not affected by my state of health. It is chronic, always with me, and I have no idea why. As a young adult I asked my family doctor if he knew what could be causing the problem. He asked me two questions. First, "Does it hurt?" and second, "Do you do anything to cause it?" My answer to both questions was an emphatic, "No, why would I?" and he changed the subject. In other words, "Just deal with it." Today I still hear sounds in my ears when I swallow, yawn, or open my mouth wide, but over time their effect has diminished and faded into normalcy. After all I have been through, dealing with this condition is easy.

I came across an interesting study conducted in 1994 by Dr. Talal

Nsouli of Georgetown University School of Medicine.[15] The research tested 100 children who had recurring ear infections. Food allergy tests revealed that about a third of them were allergic to milk and a third were allergic to wheat. Four out of five children were allergic to some type of food that was eaten on a regular basis. Parents kept these offending foods out of their diets for four months. Ear problems were strictly monitored. As a result of these dietary changes, seven out of ten children showed significant improvement. The foods were then re-introduced, and within four months, 94 percent had a recurrence of fluid build-up in their ears.

To me, this study (among many others) indicates that allergy (particularly food allergy) should at least be considered when investigating ear problems. Sadly, this is not always the case. Congestion and swelling in the nasal passages, throat, and Eustachian tube are contributing factors as well. The reason for ignoring the possibility of allergy is a mystery to me. Earaches are unbelievably painful, especially for children. Pain medicine, antibiotics, and tubes are not the best, and should not be the only, answer.

One year when our children were in elementary school, Michael and I were co-presidents of the Glenwood PTA. Our major spring fundraiser was a huge spaghetti supper in the school cafeteria. It was successful, and we made a lot of money for the school. I was sick for the entire two weeks while we directed the project. I was very good at hiding my symptoms, but what started out as my familiar seasonal allergies quickly spread to both my ears. Non-steroidal anti-inflammatory drugs eased the pain for a while, but soon both my ears were completely stopped up and I could not hear a thing.

I dreaded going to the doctor because the medicines made me feel even worse and so drowsy I would not be able to function. There was no way I would leave Michael to manage everything by himself. Over-the-counter meds were even worse. Luckily that evening the cafeteria was noisy and crowded so everyone had a hard time hearing. Michael and I worked out a series of signals, but it was difficult

---

15 Annals of Allergy 73(3), 2015-2019, 1994

to direct such a huge project when I had no idea what anyone was saying. I just smiled and we did the best we could. By the end of the evening my ears were ringing and my head was pounding.

When everything was cleaned up (we, of course, were the last to leave) I went home and slept for 16 straight hours. The fluid build-up was a breeding ground for bacteria, and in my experience, this condition never cleared up on its own. Another round of antibiotics and other medicines was necessary and I spent the next three weeks in bed. Had I been immunized or at least participating in an allergy treatment program, none of this would have happened. I have learned a lot about "allergy ears." I was suffering in silence, which proves that allergy can delve much deeper than one might think. Had I been sniffling and sneezing, exhibiting the outward signs, I obviously would not have been serving spaghetti to the public, but now I know that silent allergy symptoms can be more serious than a sneeze.

When I went off to college in 1965, pierced ears were suddenly all the rage. Girls were sterilizing needles with fire and alcohol and jabbing holes in each other's earlobes. As a result, many ears were becoming itchy, painful, swollen, and infected. Mine were no exception. I dealt with painful leaky blisters for several weeks. After diligently swabbing my ears with rubbing alcohol and peroxide, I finally gave in to the realization that pierced ears were not to be part of my fashion statement. I gave up.

Later in my allergy research I learned about nickel allergy. Piercing was not the problem. It was the nickel in the apparatus, the backings, and the earrings themselves. I eventually went to my doctor and he pierced my finally-healed ears with a stainless-steel needle. I could only wear nickel-free, gold, sterling silver or stainless steel earrings, including the backings. They were hard to find and usually expensive, but worth it because my ears were no longer infected.

Even though nickel-free earrings for sensitive ears are now more readily available and less expensive for the customer, the backings, wires and posts are not necessarily nickel-free. I highly recommend that you be cautious and exercise due diligence if you are an allergic consumer or if you are shopping for one. Other types of jewelry and watches can also contain nickel, and the content is not always noted on the tags. Nickel-free piercing guns are also making their way into the market. Although becoming de-sensitized or immunized to nickel or other metals is not yet possible, my extreme reactions have become much less severe. Perhaps I am more tolerant now, as the piling on factor plays a less predominant roll in my life. Whenever necessary, I dip the posts into hydrocortisone anti-itch cream or rub some on my earlobes for clip-on style. Now I can even wear my heirloom vintage jewelry with no problems, and that is a very good thing indeed. Grandma would be proud!

HANDWRITING ON THE WALL
#allergychangesmycalligraphytochickenscratch

Some of us are blessed with beautiful artistic handwriting while others can barely manage a little chicken scratching. Penmanship is not usually related to allergy, but it can make a difference for people like me. During my most allergified years, my handwriting could change dramatically from day-to-day, week-to-week, and even hour-to-hour or sentence by sentence. Through the years I have journaled copious pages of facts and feelings regarding my ever-changing state of allergification. In these journals my penmanship runs the gamut from calligraphy grade to barely readable and bizarre. Perfectly formed cursive letters give way to child-like printing on the same page. There are words and sentences slanting far-left and far-right. Some letters are extra-small, some are extra-large, and sometimes a page appears as just a mish-mash of assorted messy styles.

I am not talking about careless handwriting as a result of being tired or in a hurry. That experience is common for everyone. As an artist, I can design a style if I choose. These journal pages had nothing to do with artistic expression. Far from it. Changing styles were never on purpose, but clearly the most unusual handwriting examples occurred as I tried to record my most frustrating and unusual allergic experiences, often while in the throes of an extreme reaction. The quality of my penmanship (or lack thereof) was clearly related to the monsters in my system. To me, these journalistic patterns to are undeniably linked to my other ongoing symptoms at the time.

In the early 1990's when I became healthy enough to attain my Montessori degree, my huge notebook containing all my submitted tests and essays is filled with pages of beautiful, unchanging cursive manuscripts. The difference between these pages and those in my early journals is truly remarkable.

Dysgraphia refers to a condition in which a person has difficulty with written expression. It comes from the Greek word dys, meaning impaired, and graphia, meaning making letter forms by hand. It is a brain-based issue, not the result of a child or adult being lazy. I believe my penmanship changes occurred when allergens affected my brain. I had similar issues with mild temporary aphasia. In the midst of a strong allergic reaction, I would find myself struggling to find a word. Obviously, since I am an author, these conditions are now nonexistent. They disappeared along with all my other allergy symptoms.

Even still today there are graphologists (experts who study handwriting) who claim that they can predict a person's personality and behavior traits based on the size, formation, and slant of a handwriting sample. They use handwriting to identify the very essence of the person who produced it. If this is true, I must have at least ten or twenty different essences, based on which example is submitted! In actuality, the scientific community debunked this theory long ago.

I am not saying that allergy causes changes in penmanship. I am saying that in some cases observing temporary changes in penmanship could offer a clue to an otherwise undetected allergic condition, especially in children. For me, when allergy was involved on a significant level, my pencil seemed to have a mind of its own. Why would I choose to scribble rather than write legibly? Sometimes I just didn't have the energy to hold the pencil correctly. The important thing was managing to get my words on paper. I could decipher it later.

Dr. Doris Rapp, pediatric allergist and author, has written a book entitled *Handwriting Can Reveal Allergies*[16] in which she discusses the link between penmanship and allergies. Her observations deal mainly with children but can relate just as well to adults. I am a prime example. I am convinced that in addition to the body and brain, allergy can have a strong impact on motor skills.

As a teacher, I observed changes in handwriting related to other physical and emotional changes in my students. It was difficult, if not impossible, to get staff, parents, or anyone else to take me seriously. "She's just not trying," they would say. Maybe so, but there could be an underlying reason why that is the case. I am convinced that environmental exposure and diet should always be considered as a contributing factor to these otherwise unexplainable handwriting issues.

One young boy in my class always struggled with concentration and handwriting immediately after lunch. The same issues did not appear to cause him problems in the morning. I convinced his parents to have him tested for allergy, and sure enough, he was allergic to several foods, especially wheat, peanuts, milk and bananas. These were among his favorite foods and were included in his lunchbox nearly every day. A few dietary changes made a big difference. He became much more alert, his handwriting and art work improved, and he was a happier child. Several years later, his parents thanked me for alerting them to his food allergies and for referring them to Dr. Pienkowski. They said their son's cursive writing had become a work of art.

The observation of handwriting variations can be a helpful tool in determining if a troubled child (or adult, for that matter) is allergic to something in the environment, or if the condition is related to a brain dysfunction. Early recognition can be very helpful in either case. I didn't make my personal handwriting connection to allergy until years after I became immunized, so it was not part of my original diagnosis and cure. Had I known then what I know now, it probably would have been.

---

16   Dr. Doris Rapp, Handwriting Can Reveal Allergies, publisher unknown

Hair and Scalp
#popularproductsproduceprettyhairanditchyflakytenderheaded-scalp

From early childhood I have endured episodes of a red, itchy, sore, flaky scalp. At one time the doctor prescribed a medication called selsun. It came in a large brown glass bottle and it smelled terrible. My mother would carefully work it into my scalp, scraping with a comb. I had to sit still without touching it for five minutes, and then she would rinse it out with cool water. The procedure felt like torture to a young child, and it never really did any good. I felt as if sometimes the application even made matters worse, but we kept on trying, just the same. Later on when they came out with Selsun Shampoo, it was actually a little helpful, but that familiar odor, though less distinct, was anything but pleasant.

I was always tender-headed and I hated having my hair combed. Aunt Lula would patiently, slowly, gently comb through my tangled curls, offering a nickel every time she pulled. I loved her, and nickels could buy a lot of things back then, but it still hurt. As a teenager I hated beauty parlors. The strong smell of permanent wave solution, "bluing," and hair sprays made me feel strange and dizzy. I dreaded having to go pick up my grandmother from her weekly appointments. She insisted I come in and "talk to the girls." Everyone thought my reluctance was because I was afraid that one of the beauticians might want to touch my hair. I couldn't convince them otherwise.

As the years went by, I came up with a solution which allowed me to avoid beauty salons altogether. I taught myself how to cut and style my own curly hair. I slept with a head full of huge orange juice can curlers every night, slicked down with a layer of "Dippity-Do" setting lotion, which reminded me of bright blue shimmering Jell-O in a jar. My friends and family were convinced that I was causing some sort of brain trauma, but somehow I learned to get a good night's sleep.

The issue of painful flaky dandruff stayed with me for a very long time. In my early twenties, Michael gave me a beautiful authentic Maui Divers pink coral ring. He had secretly saved up for it for a long time, and it was a special gift for our first anniversary. Once I forgot to take it off when I used the smelly selsun stuff and within a few minutes the pink coral was completely dissolved. I was devastated, and I still miss it. If I had known then what I know now, I might still have my ring.

Looking back, I can't help but wonder why no one made a connection between hair problems and hair products. It seems so logical to me now. I always had a clear complexion, and the discomfort was strictly related to my scalp. Perhaps the culprit was the ever-present bright green shampoo. I am convinced it was an allergy to an ingredient in my hair products. When I began trying and alternating different shampoos and conditioners, there was significant improvement. When I discovered the connection between dandruff and yeast, I was on a clear path. More about that later.

In my thirties, my hair was thinning. I was always sweeping up clumps of hair from the bathroom floor. Since I have figured out how to avoid the scalp monsters, the only hair not connected to my head is in my hairbrush, in normal amounts. It was a challenge, but I found the solution. I hope you can too.

In my quest for answers, I discovered a salon which advertised a new concept in safe hair products which supposedly also resulted in a healthy environment. I decided to give them a try. The air inside smelled fresh and clean and they offered organic, unscented, "all-natural" hair products. Within minutes of the first shampoo application, my scalp was on fire. They rinsed my hair for an hour, as I fought back the tears. Clearly "all-natural" and "allergy-free" are two entirely different concepts.

After that horrible experience, I was totally discouraged until a friend told me about a product line called Nioxin. I have no connection whatsoever to this company, but I have to tell you that I give them credit for developing an amazing line of healthy products. Their Cleanser and Scalp Therapy conditioner provided the answer I had been hoping for. No burning, no itching, just smiles of relief. My hair grew back, thicker and fuller, and there is no more dandruff. Not one little flake. I am not even tender-headed anymore! Bosley products work for me as well. They even have pump-bottle hair spray which allows me to avoid the aerosol cans. I cannot recommend these products because I don't have any way of knowing if a certain ingredient might trigger someone else's allergy, but if I solved my scalp problems, you can too. Nioxin or Bosley would be a very good place to start.

As you are searching for your own solutions, there are a few helpful hints I have to offer. Sometimes breathing the subtle fumes from bothersome hair residue on your pillow can cause problems the next morning. For me, exposure provided vague feelings of discomfort and lack of enthusiasm for the day. Frequently changing pillowcases is a good idea. If you wash your hair every day, it could be helpful to shampoo at night and use hair products, if necessary, in the morning. If your scalp behind the ears is often itching, it may be the hairspray or soap build-up on your eyeglasses. Rinsing your brush and comb often is also helpful, and the same for curling irons and velcro rollers. Still I find it hard to imagine that something as simple as leave-in conditioner or hairspray could create such far-reaching problems. The allergy connection, though very real, is hard to detect. I hope my clues will be of some assistance, even if all you have is dandruff.

HEADACHE
#justbecauseheadachesareinvisibledoesnotmeantheydontexist

Headaches are complicated. Over half the population suffers from them and over 150 different types have been identified. It feels as if over time I have probably encountered most of them. Not anymore. The last time I remember having a headache was a couple of years ago. It must have been a virus because several family members experienced the same thing. This seemed to rule out allergy.

Before I became symptom-free, headaches of various intensities were part of my everyday life. The most common pain was from pressure along the bridge of my nose, my forehead, and under my eyes. Sometimes it felt like a toothache. It was relentless. We now know that cells in the immune system sensitive to certain allergens release chemicals which encourage blood vessels in the head to swell, causing pain in these exact same areas.

Senior year in high school my doctor became convinced that my headaches were the result of eye problems. I was an avid reader and he attributed my headaches to "squinting" without realizing it as I read. I had an appointment with the eye doctor for a Monday morning. The previous weekend had been spent at a "house party" in someone else's home. My asthma symptoms were clearly bothering me, and my eyes were red and puffy. He prescribed glasses, but only for reading. I tried to use them, but never really noticed a difference other than the words were bigger. My vision was 20/20. Whenever I got a headache, my parents would ask if I had been wearing my glasses. The answer was probably no, so they continued to make the connection. I did not. In fact, I thought the opposite was true. The headaches made me "squint." I avoided wearing my glasses whenever I could get away with it.

When we got married and moved to Hawaii, I put the glasses away in a drawer and never used them again until I reached my fifties, when I needed them for reading. My headaches never completely went away, but their frequency and severity were less intense. Now we know that allergens in the air were much different in Hawaii than they were in Tennessee. Michael always says it was he who kissed my headaches away!

When we returned to Tennessee in 1969, I lived with mild to moderate recurring headaches for the next 20 years. They ranged in intensity from mildly pounding which were manageable to migraines with debilitating pain. I could never figure out what triggered them. One particularly popular migraine medicine was advertised as a cure for all headaches, but the one time I took it I had such a horrible reaction that it scared me from trying anything stronger than aspirin or acetaminophen ever again. Sometimes I took six tablets at a time in order to manage the pain.

One weekend in the late 1970's we designed and directed two

elaborate weddings in one weekend. Two rehearsal dinners Friday night, two ceremonies and two receptions on Saturday and clean-up on Sunday. Monday morning I couldn't get out of bed. I couldn't even open my eyes. The light was unbearable and the pain was excruciating. I was nauseated and it felt as if my head was going to explode. I was miserable for three full days. Tests showed no head trauma, no debilitating disease, no brain tumor and no explanation. My general practitioner called it a chronic condition, and said I would have to learn to live with it. I should just try to relax and not work so hard.

If you can imagine all the exposures I must have had, plus the pressures which naturally go along with such an undertaking, the allergy connection is an easy one to make. Everyone was sympathetic but they thought the stress was too much for me to handle. Again, as if I were at fault for scheduling too many events or not hiring enough help. That was not the problem, but we were clueless back then.

Michael felt fine, other than just naturally being tired from all the hard work, but nevertheless we limited our obligations from then on. I never understood why I reacted so differently, but now I know. When Dr. Pienkowski attributed my headaches to allergy, it was relief beyond measure. Suddenly, it all made sense. Swelling can occur anywhere, even in the brain. The best news of all was that it had never just been "all in my head."

The Complex Nature of Chemical Sensitivity
CHEMICAL INHALANTS

 # fumesandfragrancefloatingintheairforecastfakeforlornfeelings

Now that I have become aware of the many ways in which chemical fumes affect me, the list of identifiable culprits is extensive. We all know chemicals can be toxic, but not everyone recognizes and acknowledges the vast array of painful emotional reactions these airborne chemicals can trigger for those of us who are allergic or sensitive to them. Anyone can experience a toxic reaction. An allergic constitution is not required. You may be fortunate and non-reactive, but if you notice a sudden change in someone else's behavior, recognizing and identifying these possible chemical contributors could be life-changing for everyone involved.

Even a minor encounter, like the whiff of someone's cologne, has the ability to make me feel irritable, anxious, sad, overwhelmed, swollen, and angry. Sometimes it is a sudden reaction. My abdomen inflates like a basketball and tears begin to flow. Other times it is more gradual, feeling restless, then anxious, annoyed, and out of control. Sometimes there is a strong smell, but sometimes there is no smell at all. Allergen-bearing chemical fumes can be fragrance-free. Regardless of their composition, chemicals have the power to paralyze my progress.

Since these synthetic components can also accompany other allergies, I wasn't able to make a positive identification until my other symptoms were completely controlled and out of the picture. Once I understood what was happening, I still had to convince those around me. Doing so wasn't easy. Only when those closest to me truly understood what was happening did I find relief. The emotional burden of trying to explain and convince while in the midst of a severe reaction was overpowering. I was beyond allergified and everyone was affected. Life is better now, because my reactions can be isolated and they fade away on their own without escalating into emotional turmoil. As you begin to recognize the true relationship between allergic responses and behavior, I hope your life will take on a new beginning. I hope it doesn't take you 30 years.

Printer's ink is my most dreaded chemical monster. I know that seems odd for someone who became an author, and there is a whole section devoted to this phenomenon. There are obvious malefactors to deal with such as colognes and scented candles, but there are other examples which are much harder to identify and border on invisible. I had to give up my beloved midnight mass church services on Christmas Eve once I realized that the traditional incense caused me more trouble than just a coughing episode. The piling-on factor continued to affect me well into Christmas Day. Scented tissues were eliminated as well when I realized they were actually making my congestion even worse.

One year we had new carpet installed in our main hallway. We decided on the commercial glue-down variety because it is a high-traffic area. That was a very bad decision. I was allergic to the adhesive material, and the fumes permeated our entire home for two full weeks. We vacuumed and spread thick layers of baking soda for days but nothing worked. The adhesive was permanent. I couldn't quit wheezing and crying, but thankfully by then we understood the chemical explanation. At least no one thought I was crying because I didn't like the new carpet. I spent three nights in a local hotel. It was an expensive project. The fumes slowly went away, but I was sick for a long time.

A few years ago after we had installed our central heat and air system, I had an adverse reaction when we returned from a two-week vacation. Usually I feel really good and energetic when I return to my "familiar and healthy" air. This time was different. At first I thought I was just tired, suffering from jet lag, and getting older. I decided to check the air filters. As soon as I opened the grate, I began coughing. Soon I felt dizzy and started crying. The filters were different. Before we left home, the heating and air technician who does our yearly check-up put in temporary synthetic filters so we could pressure wash our permanent ones when we returned home. Obviously these filters were sending out unwanted fumes throughout the house. We immediately threw them away and re-installed our "safe" ones. You just never know when unwanted monsters might sneak their way into your home.

I have always thought that our allergies become worse when Michael mows the lawn. It makes sense that the pollen is stirred up and floats more densely in the air. He sneezes less when he wears a mask and I always stay inside. As my research continued and my level of immunity increased, I began to realize that the pollen monsters were not the only ones in the game. The term "aura" is defined as a distinctive atmosphere which surrounds a particular person, place, or thing. It refers to any invisible emanation, especially a scent or an odor. I have coined the term "allergic aura," and there is nothing mystical about it. It has to do with mowing the yard.

Have you ever walked down the aisle in a grocery store and smelled perfume, even though there is no one in sight? Or have you smelled smoke on someone who is not smoking? Or have you noticed the strong smells in the detergent aisle even though all the boxes and bottles are tightly shut? I call these phenomena allergic aura because although practically invisible, they are mysteriously lingering in the air and causing me (and many others who are most likely unaware) to have allergic reactions. Michael has observed that whenever a certain neighbor drives down the street with her car windows open there is a strong odor from her car deodorizer for quite some time after the car is gone. It is a bit of an oxymoron, he says. Efforts to make the air better for some make it troublesome for others.

For years my symptoms flared up whenever he came inside after mowing the yard. Along with the congestion, I would become irritable and upset, which made no sense. Why on Earth would I be unhappy when the newly mowed yard looked so pretty? I should have been happy and glad that I never even had to think about mowing it myself. I felt guilty because I did not want him to think I was unappreciative. My response remained a mystery until my treatments began to work and we could eliminate pollen as the cause. Gasoline fumes created a chemical aura which followed him around like a cloud as soon as he came inside and it often lasted for an hour or more.

Once we identified this strange piece of the puzzle, lawn mowing and other fume-related outdoor experiences became much more insignificant. We have learned how to manage this phenomenon very effectively. Before he comes in, I go to another part of the house while Michael showers and throws his clothes in the washing machine. I am blessed to be married to a kind and unselfish man who is more than willing to go to all this extra trouble. He has seen the positive results and assures me that they are well worth it. We have even found another piece to the puzzle. Further sleuthing revealed the fact that rather than the lawn mower fuel, it is actually the oil mixture added to the string trimmer which actually triggers my response. It seems that it is not the lawnmower gasoline which bothers me but the oil additive that goes into the weed eater. These two chores always go hand in hand, but now I can even be outside when he uses the mower as long as I go inside before he whacks the weeds!

One time our young granddaughter Sydney overheard me saying that even after I considered myself on the path to recovery, I still tried to avoid newly printed material, scented products, and pumping gas. She asked me, "Mimi, what is pumpkin gas?" We laughed, of course, but it made me think. Wouldn't it be fine if scientists could replace those smelly old fuels with aromatic pumpkin puree!

The superabundance of scented items which invade our lives today is truly astonishing. The composition of the air we breathe in our daily lives was different for previous generations. Natural fragrances in the past are now replaced with mostly synthetic chemicals, and in my humble opinion, most are unnecessary and fight with each other for the dominant role. Anyone who remembers the sweet smell of pure cotton bed linens after a day on a clothesline in the hot summer sun or a homemade sachet of lavender buds in the lingerie drawer will know just what I mean. The difference cannot be explained by words alone, and cannot be reproduced in an aerosol can.

Fortunately for me, I hardly ever perspire. I don't know why that is the case, but maybe allergy has something to do with it. Many people suffer from the opposite condition and can even be allergic to their own sweat. My natural dryness minimizes the need for deodorant or antiperspirant which do nothing more than lay down a layer of chemicals on delicate underarm tissue which can then be absorbed into my system. Coconut oil is a healthy alternative and works well as needed, even on a daily basis.

I had never heard the word "orris root" until it showed up as "highly allergic" on my allergy test. There was no Google in those days and research was not easy, but I finally found out that it refers to a powder derived from the roots of European iris flowers. Once important in Western herbal medicines, it is a fixative agent used to enhance the fragrance in scented candles, perfume, potpourri, face powder, shaving cream, sunscreen, toothpaste, bath salts, soap and lipstick, to name a few. It smells like violets, and it is everywhere. It is even an ingredient in certain brands of gin. Unfortunately, since it is a fragrance ingredient, there is no requirement that it be listed on labels. How was I to avoid something if I didn't know it was there in the first place? Dr. Pienkowski confirmed my dilemma.

Fortunately, more and more unscented products are appearing on the market today, and I choose them whenever I can. For example, why should we use scented trash bags to cover up the odor of smelly garbage in the kitchen? Just empty the trash on a regular basis, and the problem is solved. Simmering a piece of apple with cinnamon and vanilla makes the whole house smell wonderful, and eliminates the need for unhealthy synthetic air fresheners.

The following list of everyday scented items is far from complete, but it demonstrates how we are bombarded with unnecessary particles in the air we breathe on a constant basis. Finding one lovely fragrance to truly enjoy when almost everything competes and blends together in one big mishmash is difficult, if not impossible. There is nothing more beautiful to me than a sweet magnolia blossom, as long as it comes from a tree instead of a chemical laboratory. You can probably add even more to my list of scented items such as laundry detergent, fabric softener, shampoo, conditioner, hair spray, dishwasher detergent, body wash, shaving cream, deodorant, marking pens, lotions and creams, dish washing detergents, cleaning supplies such as bleach, ammonia, furniture polish, floor wax, window cleaners, silver polish, bathroom cleaners, disinfectants, air sprays, carpet cleaners, vacuum bags, sunscreen, baby powder, trash bags, toilet tissue, closet cedar, disposable diapers, car deodorizers, oven cleaners, candles, moth balls, facial tissues, paints (especially oil-based), paint thinner, chap stick, lubricants, dry cleaning chemicals, scented pinecones and artificial trees, shoe polish, stuffed animals, perfume, after shave, toys, and cologne.

Scented sticks designed to keep our garbage disposals smelling fresh are a hot market item these days. Consumers are urged to consider them a necessity for maintaining a healthy kitchen. Here is a novel idea: Run the disposal more often and don't allow rotten food to remain in it. Toss in a lemon peel once in a while if you like. Problem solved for free!

If there are teenagers in your family who have trouble waking up in the morning there is a possible culprit you may not have considered. If you have eliminated cell phones, night lights, late bedtimes, ongoing music, television and caffeine, there may be a component you haven't considered. It could be a scented item near the bed or perhaps it is a face buried in a heavily scented pillow. Morning cobwebs are not normal.

Grocery shopping is less troublesome for me today, now that I have figured out how to avoid certain aisles or at least limit the time I have to spend there. Not only do I try to buy unscented items, but I also purchase in quantity whenever I can so that I buy them less often. I also visit the scented aisles last, after I have done the majority of my other shopping. In the past I would be allergified by the time I made it to check-out and exhausted by the time I got home, dreading unpacking the car and putting the groceries away. No wonder I hated shopping. Avoiding these monsters is really a manageable task, once you understand and have a plan. You don't have to be allergic for your body to become overwhelmed by all these inhalants. We can be immunized for orris root, but there is no cure for chemical sensitivity. Obviously, we can't be injected with even minute amounts of chemicals. But we can lessen the severity of the reactions by lessening the load. Smart shopping is a necessary component.

Everyone knows by now that breathing fumes from second- hand smoke is unhealthy. I had a distressing episode with E-cigarettes last year. We were enjoying a vacation in Florida with friends and family. One evening we were having a wonderful time laughing, talking and playing games. I went out on the balcony for some fresh air and a couple of people were smoking the new E-cigarettes. I didn't think anything of it until my upper abdomen began to swell. A couple of minutes later my eyes filled with tears and I became visibly upset. I panicked because as usual, nothing bad had happened. I rushed to our bedroom and closed the door, hoping no one had noticed my sudden departure and change of heart. Soon Michael noticed I was missing. He opened the door and saw me sitting in the middle of the bed, crying my eyes out.

"The E-cigs got me," I said. I wanted to hide under the covers. Rather than being confused and even irritated as could have happened in the past, he opened his arms and hugged me, rubbing my back until the reaction slowly subsided. "I get it," he said, and we smiled together through the tears. Soon I was able to rejoin the crowd. I winked at Jennifer and she understood what was going on. Crisis averted, the party went on into the wee hours, and a good time was had by all.

Printer's Ink
#iwishiwerenotallergictomoney

Disputing the power of printer's ink is impossible. I am guessing that most people have never considered the following scenario. You go to the book store and buy the latest best-seller which you have been looking forward to reading. You go home and snuggle down into your favorite comfortable chair, flip through the pages and begin to read. Within moments you start to feel uncomfortable, then a little anxious, and finally, sad. Your eyes well-up with tears and you are visibly upset. The emotional quandary has nothing to do with the plot or the story line. The words blur on the page and you have no more desire to read. You can't figure out what is happening, and the situation makes you even more unhappy. Your children come in and ask what is making you cry. You say you don't know. They don't believe you. The ensuing emotional predicament escalates because they think you are keeping something from them. Soon it is a family problem. Who made Mom cry? Somebody must have said or done something wrong. Is she keeping some sort of bad news from us?

All you wanted to do was read a good book. What happened?

These are the kinds of mysterious situations which I have spent decades figuring out. In this case, I am allergic to printer's ink. I know it sounds impossible, but it is true.

The word "paperless" is one of my favorite words of all time. Bills and documents can now be delivered and paid via computer. Obsolete paper phone books can be tossed in the trash, replaced with the same information accessible online. Television and computers are an alternate source to newspapers and magazines which used to provide the daily weather and news. Junk mail can be tossed into the recycle bin before it ever enters the house.

Printer's ink has turned out to be the biggest monster I have ever encountered. The discovery of this allergic phenomenon ranks among the most important events of my life. It could not have happened if I had not been immunized. As various culprits were discovered and eliminated one by one, this single mysterious monster continued to loom large. It was always in my environment, hiding in the shadows, weaving its way in and out of my life, complicating all my attempts at puzzle-working and mystery-solving. It made me feel upset, overwhelmed and angry. It produced volumes of unwelcome tears and unexplainable extreme sadness and anger. It came out of nowhere and it remained unidentified for many long years.

You might be living in a similar situation. Your monster could be something other than printer's ink but equally illusive. Elimination is not often easy, even once you figure out the source. It could be anything. There are no rules.

Looking back, I have probably always had difficulties with ink, but for some reason my responses have increased in intensity through the years. If I had identified the problem early on, when the newspapers put me to sleep as a teenager, my life could have taken a different turn. I encourage you to look outside the box, behind the walls, and under every rock whenever something just does not seem right.

Newsprint makes my eyes burn. Back when we used to have the local paper delivered every day, my eyes would itch and water as soon as I touched it. Rubbing my eyes with fingers which had been holding the printed pages only made it worse. We lived near the printing facilities so our newspaper arrived when the print was barely even dry. At one point I came up with the idea of baking the paper in a warm oven in an attempt to dry the ink. The process helped a little with my itchy eyes, but now I know that the resulting infusion of chemical fumes into the air simply caused another problem. We eventually cancelled our subscription. From then on the news, especially local events, was difficult to follow. There was no internet. Now I know why I dreaded helping Andy to deliver his neighborhood paper route.

In my teenage years, my mother used to say to me, "Don't be so dramatic." I didn't understand what she meant at the time, but she thought I was over-reacting. I probably was. Maybe it was the Sunday paper with all the colorful comics and the daily papers that stayed around the house all week. There is no way to know for sure, but allergens were floating in the air. It was a dilemma. Confrontation was always uncomfortable for me. I avoided it most of the time, but when my emotions got out of control, I didn't know how to calm down on my own. Maybe she thought I wasn't trying hard enough, but I was. Even then I sensed that something unusual was interfering with my best efforts. It was a mystery, but for the time being I had to blame it on the unsolvable dilemma of adolescence.

There is no cure for chemical allergy. Dr. Pienkowski cannot inject ink or some other chemical into my system the same as he does with a mold spore or a grain of pollen. The point is that because my chemical reactions are no longer piling on top of all the others, I have been able to identify the problem on my own. Sometimes it still creeps up and catches me unaware, but most often I can anticipate and thus avoid the escalating factors of misunderstanding and confusion which have always exacerbated the situation. The ambush factor is something I will always have to live with until that blessed day arrives when a cure is finally found.

Most importantly, those around me understand what is going on and they accept the fact that chemicals are the monsters, and not something they have unknowingly said or done. I am no longer accused of dramatically over-reacting and for sure my loved ones know that these previously bizarre occurrences are real. Of all my discoveries, this one means the most.

One sunny afternoon Jennifer and I were sitting outside on our patio when for some reason Michael had set the fax machine on the table behind us. I had no idea it was there. All of a sudden I began to feel stressed and on the verge of tears, just sitting outside enjoying the day. The others knew I had not seen it, and it was the first real proof that ink, especially warm out-gassing ink, was the culprit. Michael removed the fax machine, and within a few minutes I was back to my smiling self. As a result, this family does not have the luxury of accompanying our computer with a printer. It is a huge inconvenience, but well worth it. Printers can emit high levels of ultrafine particles into the air. Photographs and long documents produce the most. These particles compare to those emitted by cigarette smoke and car exhaust and they have easy access to both the lungs and the brain. I can demonstrate what happens to me by intentionally causing an exposure. Proof is undeniable, and finding this gigantic piece of the puzzle is a blessing beyond belief.

A few examples of problematic sources of exposure include newspapers, books, magazines, the old ditto machines, fax machines, printers, junk mail and flyers (especially the glossy colorful pages), greeting cards, cash register receipts, stationery, business cards, instructions of all kinds, especially when emerging from their sealed plastic bags, and money, especially newly printed bills.

Before we made the connection, whenever Michael and I would sit around the kitchen table working on the budget, writing checks and managing our cash, we would often become irritated and end up fussing over some small unimportant thing. Now we know the humbug was never about our financial situation.

The printed material was causing me to feel uncomfortable, and as the monsters gradually gained strength, my attitude changed for the worse. Michael sensed the change, of course, and wondered, (often out loud), what was wrong. I didn't know, of course, and before we knew it, we were both annoyed. For the longest time, we never understood why. Now we know that without a doubt, the printer's ink was to blame.

We handle our finances differently these days. Michael does all the paper-shuffling before I even come into the room and if I start to feel uncomfortable, I just walk away for a while and he looks for hidden monsters. Electronic transactions and banking help tremendously in reducing my allergic load and we no longer have to dread monthly bill-paying sessions.

Whenever possible, I avoid visits to post offices, libraries, newspaper buildings, mail centers and book stores. This circumvention seems strange for an author, and I could never have written and published books before I figured out my allergy. To make matters even more complicated, only certain inks, not all of them, bother me. Unfortunately, there is no way to check and compare ingredients ahead of time so I just do the best I can. Severe reactions in the past prohibited me from even considering writing books, but now that I am not responding to most other things, printer's ink has become a manageable, though possibly ever-present trigger. As I have gradually attained a clearer understanding of the monster's modus operandi, I am much more qualified to defend myself. The detective in me still refuses to let the guard down.

The process of discovery was very gradual. As I became immune to dust and mold, musty old books no longer contributed to my allergies. I still wasn't comfortable spending time in libraries, and now I know that new books and recently printed periodicals are still a problem to some extent. Once they have been previously read and the pages aired out, I can manage fairly well.

I love greeting cards. I love the art work, the messages (even the corny, cheesy silly ones) and the sheer beauty of the elaborate ones. They don't like me. I especially love Christmas cards. They provided a chance to communicate with loved ones before social media took over, even if only once a year. One November Michael and I found four large boxes of beautiful expensive Victorian designer cards on sale for half price. We bought them all! I went home and made out my long list of friends and family, verified addresses, retrieved my red and green calligraphy pens and bought the perfect holiday postage stamps. Everyone would get a personal message. I pulled out our vinyl records and cassette tapes of all my favorite Christmas carols, enough to last all day. I set up my card table with everything I needed and I was filled with the Christmas Spirit. I unwrapped the plastic wrapping and carefully opened each box. I set the four piles in front of me. From then on, everything is a blur.

In the space of a few short minutes, I became sad, upset, frustrated and angry. The project was ruined, and that made me cry even more. I ended up throwing everything out the door. Boxes, cards, envelopes, stamps, and everything else scattered all over the patio. I could hardly breathe, my stomach swelled up like a basketball and I ended up crying hysterically in a heap on the floor. For the first time I heard myself sobbing, "Why is this happening to me?"

When Michael came in and saw the situation he was at a loss. He just stared at me like a deer in the headlights, having no idea what to do. In truth, there was nothing he could do. I was inconsolable. He finally got me into bed and I slept for four long hours. When I woke up I was calm, and except for the puffy eyes from all that crying, I was nearly back to normal. We hugged each other, and I assured Michael that he had done nothing wrong. I hoped he believed me. I had no explanation. He swept up the mess on the patio and threw it all in the trash. No one would hear from us that year, and for that I was legitimately sad.

The best conclusion to come out of that episode is that we finally figured out that outgassing fumes from all the elaborately printed material were responsible for my reaction. We had suspected that printer's ink was a problem but for the first time there simply was no other explanation. What to do about it was another matter entirely. It was a mystery identified but not understood, and a long way from being solved.

My allergy to ink and many other chemicals can wreak havoc

on my emotions. Yours could be affecting you in an entirely different way. Swelling can occur anywhere in the body, even in the emotional centers of the brain. There are no cookie cutter answers, but the possibilities are endless. No matter how unrealistic or unimaginable it might seem, allergy really could be the answer.

This discovery opened up a whole new list of possible explanations for me. The Christmas card episode was extravagant, but often my reactions, though real, were much more subtle in nature. I began to realize that changes in my moods really did have a physical explanation. It was not just all in my head, and it was not preventable. Understanding what was happening was the first step. Convincing others would prove to be more difficult. It took time.

From then on, I was determined to find out what was really going on. I connected opening gifts and packages, wrapping paper, greeting cards, bubble packs, instructions sealed in plastic, receipts, and other special occasion items to my list of miscreants. Tossing holiday wrapping paper into the fireplace and burning newspapers, even in the outside fire pit, were problematic. Scented markers and other toys and even opening new decks of playing cards could release fumes which my confused immune system identified as hazardous. Sometimes I could keep track of almost every card in a hand of bridge. Other times I needed a review of the bidding. No one ever suspected a new deck of cards. Now we know. You can see from these few examples that my senses were challenged on special occasions. Some people are not particularly fond of parties, games, gifts, and other celebrations. I am not one of them. Controlling my dreaded negative reactions on special occasions was one of the hardest things I have ever had to do. I am now a consistently average bridge player.

As we figured out ways to prevent the printer's ink from invading my environment, I began to feel better on a consistent basis. The "thick air" as I called it, was becoming thinner, and friends and family were coming on board. I was on my way to a symptom-free life, and a few little chemicals were not going to wreak any more emotional havoc.

We gradually learned how to clear the air. We open all the mail outside and discard it when possible. We mounted an "air-out basket" (the AOB) outside the kitchen door so that printed material which must come inside can remain there until the ink evaporates. We go "paperless" at every opportunity. We cancelled all newsletter and magazine subscriptions. This decision was a hard one, but the monsters left us no choice. The pretty glossy pages could no longer live in our house. These days I sometimes spend extra time in various waiting rooms because the older well-read magazines are not a problem. I have even been known to sit back down in the lobby after my appointment to continue reading an interesting article! The invention of the Kindle and e-books has made a big difference in my life.

Even in health-related magazines and other periodicals, I seldom see any reference to chemical allergy, especially a printer's ink problem. Avoiding the subject makes sense from their point of view, I guess, because magazines and newspapers would hesitate to print such informational articles for fear of losing customers. This financial philosophy is something worth thinking about.

Once we became aware of the allergy connection, those who love me take their gifts out of the manufacturer's sealed packaging and re-wrap them after they air out. We take the Christmas wrapping paper and empty boxes outside as soon as possible after the gifts are opened. In the past I loved to see the mounds of boxes, paper, ribbons and bows all over the floor around the tree, adding to the festivity of the morning. Now we know better. Holiday joy is so much more than paper and bows. Cards are opened outside before bringing them in to post around the door. I guess I should be glad that printed greetings are being replaced by digital messages, but I do miss the charm of pretty paper cards.

Once my Aunt Pellen gave me a brand new paperback copy of *The Thorn Birds*. I journaled this episode long before I made the ink connection. I was always a calm, quiet, laid-back sort of person, but not on the day when I decided to read that book. I had always loved to read, but this time something made me lose my temper. Someone said something to me (I have no idea what), and I threw the book all the way across the dining room. It stayed there on the floor for a very long time. If I picked it up, it was an admission that I threw it. The rest of the family left it there as a monument to the fact that I really did throw it. I eventually picked up the book and read it, probably long after the ink had dried on the pages. It is one of my all-time favorites, and today it is prominently displayed in our bookcase as a great reminder of just how far we have come. The amazing flying book!

Our grandson Joshua is very protective of me, and he is very attentive to anything coming inside which could cause a problem for his Meems. Once we bought him an expensive Lego set and he couldn't wait to sit down on the floor with me and put it together. By the time we opened all the little plastic bags and spread out the instruction sheets, I was wheezing and tearing up and we had to stop until the fumes were gone. He was so kind and understanding at that young age. I marvel at the concept of how wonderful it is that children are often the first ones to truly "get it." My heart warms, just knowing that this awareness is being passed on to future generations.

WATER (H2O)
#waterwatereverywherebutwhatamitodrink

Water is, after all, just chemicals. There is a term for water allergy. It is called aquagenic urticaria or aquagenic pruritis. It refers to a rash caused by contact with water. I have never experienced a water rash, but I have wondered on occasion if I might be allergic to my own tears. Perhaps the water composition in our bodies changes naturally from time to time. My reactions are puzzling. One thing is certain, however. There is never any shortage of water in my tear ducts and the spigots turn on at the least provocation. Every time I yawn, water flows. I yawn a lot. Sometimes my eyes itch and burn as a result. Sometimes they don't. I blamed my make-up until journaling discounted the connection. I have alternated brands, used one item such as mascara exclusively and I have washed away every trace. The same procedure applies to lotions and creams, both on my hands

156

and on my face. Sometimes I have a reaction and sometimes I don't but tears are always the trigger. The most intense discomfort is at the very corners of my eyes beside my nose. Every emotional experience opens the flood gates. I even cry at television commercials.

On the opposite side, I hardly ever perspire. There have been times in the earlier allergic days when I would easily become flushed and sweaty even when I was not out in the heat. Sometimes it happened in the middle of the night or in combination with another allergic reaction. It doesn't happen anymore. As a child I remember smiling when my great-grandmother Mama T, who always smelled like soft lilacs or lavender, would tell me, "horses sweat, men perspire, and women suffer from the heat." I guess she would be glad to know that none of those conditions apply to me.

Sweat is a dilute salt solution produced by the eccrine sweat glands. Perhaps some of my four million glands don't work well for some reason. That could help explain why I always need to keep the fans running and the indoor temperature so cool. The family used to call our house "Mimi's meat locker" because they always needed extra sweaters when I was perfectly comfortable in my tee shirt and shorts. Today I am comfortable at 72 degrees but still I seldom perspire. Anhidrosis is the term for the inability to perspire normally. What causes it has never been clearly defined. Perhaps my abundance of salty tears eliminates enough water from my body for both of them. It doesn't seem to interfere with my quality of life, but it could be different if I were an athlete or constantly engaging in strenuous activity, which I have never been able to do in the first place. The best thing of all is that I don't even need an antiperspirant!

When travelling to certain countries, people are often warned not to drink the water. I get that. Not only do different foods bother me, but different water does as well. Recently, I have read about studies which show that some drinking water can even cause food allergies, but research is sketchy. Bottled water is not my best choice, especially if the plastic bottles have been sitting out in the hot Florida sun or if they have been travelling across the country in a hot paneled truck.

There is not much I can do about this situation but water allergy is an interesting topic to consider. Years went by before I finally figured out that monsters were swimming in my drinking water.

Filtered water from our home refrigerator causes me no obvious problems but I wish I had a way of knowing how the chemically treated water affects me systemically. I am pretty sure that mystery is unsolvable, but still I am curious. We all know that staying hydrated is crucial for good health. Pale to clear urine is a good measure of this, and I take the issue very seriously.

I have come to the conclusion that distilled water is a good choice for me. The subject is controversial and I have studied it extensively. Distillation is a process whereby water is boiled until it turns to steam. The steam is then condensed and collected into a clean container. As it cools, it becomes distilled water. It is basically a method by which water is removed from the contaminants rather than the contaminants being removed from the water. The process is very efficient and it seems logical to me.

Most tap water is perfectly safe to drink. Regulations require it to fall between 6.5 and 9.5 on the pH scale. Neutral pH is 7.0, with alkaline registering higher and acidic being lower. Even the Environmental Protection Agency (EPA) standards allow "acceptable" levels of such things as lead, arsenic, radioactive particles, mercury, and so forth which are possibly problematic to those of us with chemical allergy. Just as I try to avoid additives in food, avoiding them in water seems to make sense as well. Removing toxins from my body appeals to me, and drinking pure water, hydrogen and oxygen, seems like a healthy way to accomplish my goal. In addition, most waterborne disease-causing bacteria are unable to survive the distillation process.

Distilled water itself is neutral, but as it comes into contact with carbon dioxide from the atmosphere it becomes slightly acidic. Our bodies function best when slightly alkaline. Some are concerned that beneficial minerals such as magnesium and calcium can be diminished when we drink distilled water. Soft drinks and many other processed items are made with distilled water but even so, water is not the essential source of these nutrients. A balanced diet is very capable of providing what our bodies require and healthy kidneys are very efficient in keeping minerals in perfect ratio. Of course supplements are available, but a diet rich in such things as dark leafy greens, yogurt, dark chocolate, avocado, legumes, nuts and seeds is much more delicious. If you are concerned about fluoride, it would have to be provided by an alternate source such as toothpaste because fluoride is not present in distilled water.

Distilled water is possibly beneficial to those with weakened immune systems but anyone suffering from illness should consult their physician before making a change. Distilled water seems to be working well for me, especially when travelling away from home. It is not for everyone, but I suggest you consider it, especially if you have allergies, chemical or otherwise.

How Allergy Influences Behavior and Emotion
DEPRESSION
#experiencingacertainsorrowtowhichwordsofcomfortdonotapply

Several years ago, as my brain fog and related symptoms began to diminish, I was able to put more effort toward writing my book. In the process, I made what I consider to be a significant discovery. I was re-visiting my emotional feelings regarding sadness, tearfulness, sleep disorders (either too little or too much), small tasks taking extra energy, anxiety, mood swings and anger, as well as unexplained physical conditions such as headache and back pain which had lived in my shadows for such a very long time.

One day during that time frame, as I was watching television, a commercial about anti-depression medication came on the screen. Suddenly, it dawned on me. The symptoms I had been dealing with for all those years were among the very same ones being used to describe depression. I had never considered a possible connection before, maybe because I was so caught up in attributing everything to allergy, my focus remained narrow. In addition, I had never known anyone who had been diagnosed with that disease so there was never an opportunity to compare notes and discuss challenges. Now I know that my allergy symptoms mimicked those of depression in a big way. The largest revelation of all is that all those symptoms simply evaporated on their own as my allergy monsters lost control.

For years, I labeled my time as either "Up Days" or "Down Days." I never knew, until I opened my eyes in the morning, which one I would encounter. "Up Days" were energetic and productive. "Down Days" found me counting the hours until I could go back to bed. My symptoms could last for moments, hours, days, or even longer. Uneasy feelings lingered in the background of my mind for extended periods. It was not until my allergies were completely under control that my "Up Days" far outnumbered the "Downs."

Feelings of sadness are normal reactions to sad events. That is not what we are talking about here. By the Grace of God, I have never experienced a cataclysmic crisis in my life. There have been times, however, when I have felt just as distraught as if something awful had actually happened.

Michael remembers times when we would be laughing together one minute and I could walk into another room and return feeling upset and unhappy about something. No words had been spoken and no one else was in the house. How could that be? My moods could change with the blink of an eye, and I was a handful. Jennifer once said to me, "Mom, a lesser man probably would have left you." She was right, but love and faith kept us together.

I have heard it said that women like to talk about our problems and men like to solve them. Of course these days we know it is not a gender issue, yet it is true that women generally speak 20,000 words per day while men speak only 7,000. In the early days, when I first realized that allergy was to blame for almost everything, Michael was not so easily convinced. He was always looking for another answer, something more concrete, carved in stone, medically explainable and acceptable. The mood swings would be easier to understand if we could prove a physical component. There was none. I just kept talking. He needed more time to accept Dr. Pienowski's spot-on diagnosis, but today he is completely on board with the notion that "all my symptoms were allergy-related."

There were times when hosting family get-togethers and celebratory occasions was a difficult task for me. I loved the festivity and sharing special recipes and traditions with all the generations. Setting the table with candles, good china, crystal, polished silver and beautiful flowers brought me joy. At first. But more often than not, I managed to feel upset, overwhelmed, and even tearful at some point throughout the process of preparing and presenting the meal. Sometimes, no one knew. Sometimes they were all aware. I always knew, but I didn't know why and I didn't know how to fix it, until now. Clearly an army of allergens was invading the air, and attacking my brain.

Onions stand out as one of the strongest uninvited monsters which chose to make an appearance at these gatherings, and I have learned a lot about them through the years. For example, I have discovered that although onions are delicious, the black residue that sometimes appears on their skin provides a breeding ground for mold. Peeling yellow onions with even a tiny bit of that common black powder on the skin could actually make me cry. These tears were different from the watery eyes we all experience from the fumes. These tears came from some form of artificial, yet at the same time very real, sadness and frustration. Mold spores, even 24 hours after exposure, had the ability to turn my emotions upside down and hurl a nice family dinner into turmoil.

My grandmother once told me that when she was a little girl, doctors placed raw onion halves, cut side up, in dishes around a sick person's bed. The idea was that the onions would absorb the germs (bacteria) in the air, thus removing sickness from the environment. Whether or not these onions were helpful in that regard is debatable, but according to her, the onions all turned black. I learned something from her onion story. The inner layers of black-skinned onions probably have the ability to absorb mold from the outer skin. If you are allergic, it would be best to avoid the black-skinned ones and throw them away. I am also careful not to leave cut onions out on the kitchen counter for a long time. They are safer from invasion in a covered dish inside the refrigerator.

Of course, onions were only part of the story of my depressing reactions to everyday items and events. I longed for the time when I could control the elusive mood swings. Regarding these special family occasions, my feelings of sadness and regret lingered long after everyone went home. Love held us together, but it could have been better. Someone else could have peeled the onions.

Now that immunotherapy has stopped my dreaded depression monsters dead in their tracks, there are only a few remaining triggers which still have the power to bring me to tears. They are basically chemical in nature and we will discuss this phenomenon as my story unfolds. I am so thankful that these allergenic exposures no longer escalate into emotional upheaval, and I have learned how to smile through the tears.

Although depression is a serious mood disorder, to me it is a vague term, more than occasional sadness, and hard to define as a disease. I read somewhere that allergic people become sad and depressed because congestion, sleepiness, and headache interfere with their daily routines, causing the "allergy blues." This simplistic insinuation that these feelings are "all in the head" must have been spoken by someone who is not allergic, because the theory is both hurtful and wrong. Coping skills can never replace a cure, and as far as I know, sneezing doesn't cause depression.

In my experience, even well-intentioned encouraging advice can have the opposite effect. Words like, "Just try and get over it" and "Things are really not so bad," can be perceived as hurtful to the person who is feeling trapped by a sense of melancholia. Of course I was trying to overcome both my feelings and my reactions to them, and becoming defensive only made matters worse. To many people, the idea that dust, food, mold, animals, and chemicals could lead to feelings of depression is a crazy concept. They are wrong. Even though I am now protected from those original evil monsters, I can still demonstrate an authentic, upsetting, tearful reaction by experiencing a legitimate encounter with one of my chemical allergens.

I have thought a lot about Seasonal Associative Disorder, also known as SAD. Apparently, people report feelings of depression which begin in late autumn, escalate through the winter, and disappear in the spring. Similar complaints linked to summer can also occur, but they are less frequent. To qualify for a SAD diagnosis, the onset and lifting of depressive episodes must be linked to a specific time of year for the previous two straight years. I feel confident that my situation matches these requirements to a certain extent.

From my perspective, if allergy were to be considered as a contributor, treatment could begin immediately after testing, and the two years of suffering from the symptoms could be at least partially alleviated much sooner. I never connected myself with the term SAD because my symptoms intermingled and I could not determine a beginning and an end. Singling out and treating them one by one was impossible because they refused to stand in line. I owe my emotionally stable and happy life to Dr. Pienkowski and his determination to treat my whole body as a combination of symptoms and events. As I continue to try and gain more information about suggested causes and treatment for SAD, one word is conspicuously absent from all my reading. That word, of course, is allergy.

According to the Mayo Clinic[17], the specific cause of SAD is unknown. They suggest that several factors, such as disruption of your biological clock (circadian rhythm), lower serotonin levels (related to decreased sunlight), and disruption in melatonin levels (which affects sleep patterns and mood) could be responsible for the melancholia. Lower levels of Vitamin D attributed to sunlight deficiency is listed as a possible contributing factor as well.

Suggested treatments include lightbox therapy, medication, behavioral therapy, more exercise, meditation, stress management techniques, mental health assessments, and visiting climates that offer more sunshine. Merchants are jumping on the bandwagon, offering many types of lightboxes, from designer styles to medical grade

---

17 www.mayoclinic.org

equipment with best price and most reliability. I understand that increased light can be beneficial to lots of people, but all this hoopla makes no sense to me. If someone suggested that in order to cure my feelings of depression, I should go work out at the gym, it would border on insulting. I have another idea.

Many environmental changes occur as we approach the winter months. We turn on the furnace for the first time and accumulated dust and allergens fly through the ductwork and bombard the air. Gas heat is especially troublesome for many unsuspecting people. We light up the fireplace logs or turn on the gas-fed ones. We cuddle under woolen blankets previously stored in moth balls or in grandmother's lovely cedar chest. We bring out the goose-down or feather-filled comforters which are packed away again in the spring. We bring down dusty old holiday decorations from the musty attic or from a damp corner in the basement. We fill our homes with winter greenery and scented candles. We close our windows so indoor allergens are even more concentrated. Pets spend more time indoors than out, and the list goes on…

Sometimes my sniffles and sneezes escalated with the spring grasses and pollen, and then lessened through the summer. Categorizing my various symptoms by season was difficult because so many of them never went away. For someone less allergic, the seasonal differences could tend to be more obvious. I am just offering another avenue for those suffering from SAD (as well as other issues of depression) to explore.

Millions of Americans cope with feelings of despondency every day and in many cases, modern medicine is yet to find a cure. I endured many such symptoms for decades and I do not have them now. I never spent a moment in psychotherapy and there was never a regimen of anti-depressant medication. Those sad feelings are now only distant memories. Immunotherapy provided my cure.

A short while ago, I was enjoying a conversation with a friend of mine, a member of the clergy. We were discussing my upcoming book, and my intense determination to make not only an emotional appeal for more understanding about the role allergy can play in our lives, but hopefully a significant medical contribution as well. We discussed the fact that I believe God brought us through these years in order to make a difference for others. He told me that in all his years (and he is approaching retirement) of counselling parishioners, he had never made the connection between allergy, emotional well-being, behavior, and pain. He appreciates his newfound compassionate insight and looks forward to using my story as he counsels others in their quest for peace.

ANGER ISSUES
#unprovokedangryoutburstsareawful

There is nothing in my simple life to make me feel angry. I am by nature a quiet loving person. I am also human. I get annoyed by certain issues, especially political and social ones. I get frustrated when I encounter situations out of my control. I get upset when I perceive injustice and criminal misbehavior makes me angry. It is emotionally healthy to experience and express anger when justified. Cause and effect is a logical concept. Unexplainable angry outbursts and over-reactions are another matter entirely.

I have finally discovered that certain chemical exposures can trigger in me sudden intense feelings of anger and rage when there is absolutely no perceived threat or provocation. They are totally spontaneous and can be extreme beyond allergified. I know this concept defies common theories, but it happens to me and I can demonstrate it by an intentional exposure. Reactions can also be less severe and they can escalate.

The left temporal lobe is the part of the human brain associated with temper control. Certainly some reaction could be expected whenever this area becomes swollen or inflamed. I don't understand why it is not considered as a possible cause of angry feelings by anyone else but me. Swelling can occur anywhere. In my general research allergy is completely ignored as a possible contributing factor. My goal is to offer my discovery as a very real explanation for others to consider. Recently a young person, age 12, confided an interesting scenario. He said he was walking by himself down the hall at school. It was crowded, between classes. He was suddenly overwhelmed with a strong feeling of anger. He had no idea what caused it and it had never happened to him before. It was disturbing, of course, but it didn't last long. This child is a well-adjusted, happy straight-A student. The feelings came out of nowhere, and I wonder if perhaps it was something from the chemistry lab, or maybe a teacher's cologne. We don't know of course, but if these angry feelings suddenly descended upon a troubled child, the scenario could potentially turn out much differently. I am simply offering this observation to raise awareness about the possibilities.

Before I realized what was happening to me in these situations, I was at a loss. How do you explain to your husband and children that even though you feel angry, you really are NOT angry? The task is impossible to accomplish in the moment. As I felt these emotions building up, sometimes I would try to avoid any confrontation by escaping to my bedroom. It only made matters worse. Of course they didn't understand, and I was accused of running away to avoid taking responsibility for my "temper tantrums." Thank goodness my anger never progressed beyond words.

My angry episodes were much less prevalent than my tears, but when they occurred they presented a real struggle for me. There was no way to avoid guilty feelings for causing problems even though I would never intentionally cause any hurt feelings or misunderstandings on purpose. I was responsible for my behavior even though I had no idea what to do about it. There is a difference between an excuse and an explanation. I make no excuse but I am so glad we finally have an explanation.

As a result, these angry monsters only make an appearance once in a while, and now that we know what invites them, they don't have much power over me at all. Reducing their power wasn't possible because I was in such a highly allergic state. Piling on made the situation even worse. When we examine the circumstances there is always an allergen around. I try to stay calm and ignore the anger monsters and my family understands. I wish that were true for other victims. If these frustrating allergy-related angry outbursts can happen to me, surely others are vulnerable as well. I believe these sudden, unwelcome feelings of anger can happen to anyone at any age.

My brother and I remember evenings in our youth when our parents would get mad at each other, bicker and fuss over small things which seemed to us trivial and unimportant. The next morning they behaved as if nothing had happened. We were never given an explanation, probably because there was none. They loved each other, but I believe they both must have been allergified by the end of the day. This understanding on my part came too late for me to share it with them, but I am certain that had we known back then what we know today, immunization would have given my parents many more happy hours.

Allergic reactions could be playing a much bigger role than we imagine in cases of road rage, domestic issues, childhood misbehavior and various social confrontations.

Of course my opinions are modestly unprofessional, and based only on my own personal experiences, but I truly believe that mental health professionals could benefit immensely by devoting more attention to the allergy factor. Surely I am not the only person whose anger issues have always been allergy-related. It is so important for anger management courses to take this subject very, very seriously. Those who are prone to violence are at an even greater risk. Enough said.

ADDICTION
#cravingscreateaconstantquandary

Addiction comes in many forms, not just street drugs, medications and alcohol. I have never been addicted to alcohol or anything illegal, but I do believe I am addicted to food. It is something that no matter how hard I try, I cannot do without. Food consumption complicates my life in a lot of ways. Addiction is an intricate and complex concept and it reaches far beyond familiar associations.

I smoked cigarettes for a few years, beginning in college when it was fashionable and "the thing to do." I was hooked from my first cigarette. I was probably already addicted from living in a home filled with second-hand smoke from the day I was born. My body was already craving the nicotine. On the other hand, my younger brother never smoked. Perhaps he never even tried, and that is how he avoided that terrible habit. Maybe he didn't inherit the severe allergic constitution which has been my companion for all these years. Modern science has no answer and neither do I, but I wonder.

In an effort to combat my lingering post-pregnancy obesity, my doctor prescribed diet pills which were legal and popular at the time. I quickly lost 60 pounds. We now know that they were powerful amphetamines, and without really understanding what their possible long-term effects could mean, I was addicted. After the weight loss, I soon realized that I was relying on them for energy, and for an unknowing allergic young mother, it was welcome assistance. Thankfully I realized that I did not want to go down that path, no matter how tempting the prospect was to help keep the monsters at a distance. After several long months I gave them up cold-turkey and after a couple of weeks I felt better. Even when my weight began to slowly return, I never considered anything like that again. I often longed for an "energy shot," but drugs are not the answer. I believe God was protecting me for a higher purpose.

Years later, working in the flower shop, depression reared its ugly head. My family doctor, who was also a good family friend, prescribed Elavil, a tricyclic antidepressant. It had no effect. He then prescribed Valium. Again, recognizing the addictive possibilities, I put it in my dresser drawer "for later, just in case I really need it." I never did take it. Even back then, somehow I knew that something else was going on. Even as a renowned and respected diagnostician, his training couldn't solve my mysteries. Once he reluctantly offered to get me into the Koala Center, the mental health wing of Oak Ridge Hospital, hoping maybe one of the great minds there might offer some insight.

He was going to sneak me in through the private back door because he really didn't think I belonged there. He was running out of answers on his own. I appreciated his care and concern, but I did not go. I toughed it out, not wanting medication to mask the symptoms and destroy the clues. Without the loving support of family, who understood even less than I did, it would have been easy to choose a path of lifelong dependence.

Since my youth I have always felt that I have addictive tendencies. Maybe it is genetic, because many people do not have similar feelings which help them recognize the caution flag in their early years. My mother's father, a wonderful man who was wealthy, generous, and well-loved by all who knew him, was an alcoholic. He died of cirrhosis of the liver when I was only four years old. His gift is that I have always been careful not to let that happen to me. Many people enjoy a cocktail at the end of the day to help them relax, change their mood or perk them up. That's why they call it Happy Hour. Alcohol does not have that effect on me. I am fortunate that I did not drink excessively in an effort to help alleviate my allergy symptoms. I was borderline drowsy so much of the time already. I would have a "social drink" and nurse it along, just to join in the festivities, but truth be told, it might just as well have been a pretty glass of water.

Some people do believe there is a connection between allergy and alcohol addiction. It could be the yeast, the additives, the processing procedure or even the corn in the bourbon or the potatoes in the vodka. Since most ingredients are not on the label, detective work is limited in that regard.

My daddy always enjoyed a can of beer, especially Budweiser, but something happened whenever he drank a can of Schlitz. One time after a couple of sips, he sneezed 17 times in a row. We counted! He absolutely refused to say that he was either addicted or allergic to beer. Now we know that the problem was something much more specific than just "beer." My point is that rather than give it up entirely if you have a problem, you might first explore the notion of changing brands.

I have heard people say that they believe someone is allergic to beer or alcohol. Neither of these words refers to a single ingredient. "Beer belly" is just a general term and there are many alternatives to explore before giving up alcohol altogether. Perhaps it is an allergy (or maybe even an addiction) to an ingredient such a hops, barley, brewer's yeast, or any other item found in a particular brand. Severe Oak tree allergy could be a problem with bourbon processed and stored in oak casks. Even the smell of bourbon used to make me feel sick. Sugar could be a problem if you drink rum or it could be something in the mixer with which it is combined. Both allergy and addiction are complicated issues but more and more studies are being conducted in search of connections and cures. Your personal detective work could be well worth the effort in the meantime. In the old days, American beer was just hops, water, and barley. Recipes are more complicated today, and often kept secret, but sometimes lists of ingredients are readily available in craft beer, especially if the beverage is produced locally.

I do think that in my own way, I am addicted to one particular libation. As newlyweds, Michael and I went to visit his sweet little white-haired Aunt Mabel in Asbury Park, New Jersey. Sitting in her beautiful Victorian parlor, I began to suffer with female monthly discomfort (a subject one did not discuss in polite society in those days). She sensed what was going on and offered me a nice glass of her best Blackberry Brandy. That was 1969. It actually did the trick with no side effects and turned out to be far superior to a Midol addiction. To this day, I do enjoy raising a glass in a toast to Aunt Mabel from time to time. If this is an addiction, it is a good one.

My favorite prescription cough syrup produced a feeling of euphoria, so I would take only the tiniest sip when nothing else would work. Coughing was so much a part of my life that I could have easily given in and depended on constant doses all day long. Dr. Pienkowski came to the rescue and replaced my codeine with better, non-addicting cough suppressants which really worked.

Along with my diagnosis of food allergy came the notion that cravings for specific foods can play an important role in managing or not managing allergies. The idea is that quite often if you either love or hate a certain food, you may be allergic to it. As a child, the only food I did not like was carrots, especially cooked ones. They made me shiver. I doubt it was mere coincidence that my first food allergy test showed that I was highly allergic to carrots. Otherwise, I enjoy all kinds of foods and trying to avoid those on my list was quite a challenge. In my mind, I was and I still am severely addicted to certain foods, especially carbohydrates. And green beans.

When people speak of food addiction, it usually pertains to sweet and salty junk food, fast food, and highly processed foods. I rarely eat these things anymore, but my brain remembers. Driving by places like Krystal, McDonalds, and Krispy Kreme Donuts without experiencing at least a small urge to pull in to the drive-thru has always presented a real challenge. I read somewhere that the proteins in some foods contain heroin-like peptides which could perhaps contribute to severe cravings in susceptible individuals. There is no way to know for certain, but I am pretty sure I fit in that category. Although less intense and better understood, the urges remain and on occasion I give in to them. I am human, after all.

My final diagnosis was hard to comprehend. I am allergic to almost everything I eat. I was completely overwhelmed. What was I to do? As I said before, an alcoholic can give up alcohol, and a drug addict can give up drugs, but giving up food is impossible. This was the biggest mystery of all. If I avoid a certain food, my allergy to it diminishes. But when I do eat it, I become allergic again and the cycle continues. The connection to addiction is undeniable.

Fortunately, my condition is rare. I don't wish for a stomach ache or a rash, but at the same time if I had some sort of signal, it might help me to better understand the nature of this allergy. Instead, my symptoms are hidden systemically, adding to my general allergic state. I am also addicted to the process of trying to manage my foods, making sure I have healthy choices on hand and planning as much as possible so I don't get caught by surprise. If I were only dealing with a few foods, keeping track by journaling would be well worth the effort. In my situation it would be a monumental task. These days since I am symptom-free in other areas, food management for me has become more of a choice than a necessity. If there is such a thing as a "foodaholic," I fit the category very well. Had I not been tested for food allergy, I believe I would still be unaware of my condition.

Lots of people claim an addiction to coffee, tea, soft drinks, energy drinks or other sources of caffeine. Billions of people around the world enjoy a cup of coffee every morning. Others avoid these drinks at all cost because of severe allergic reactions. During my most intense allergy years, caffeine had no effect on me. I longed for a midday pick-me-up but even a huge cup of expresso with sugar and cream did little more than taste good. My monsters were in control and ignoring caffeine was their mantra.

These days I can enjoy a cup of coffee or tea in the afternoon, and it gives me the same energy boost that most people get with their morning cup. I have never re-developed any kind of dependency on coffee (if I had one in my earlier years), and I think my current state of good health is responsible. I wonder if the mycotoxins (mold) often present in coffee could have caused drowsiness to counteract the caffeine before I was immunized. My body's up and down secretions of the hormone cortisol could possibly effect my energy levels and their relationship to caffeine, but the theory of a genetic component doesn't seem to apply here because of the inconsistency in my responses. The reason why some people react to caffeine and others do not remains a medical mystery.

I have reached one conclusion that I adamantly believe to be true. Food addiction is not about a lack of willpower. It is caused by the intense dopamine signal that "highjacks" the brain's biochemistry. It is very real to me. The term, "all things in moderation" sounds good and may work well for lots of people, but not for me. There is more about the carbohydrate connection and cravings later in the book.

I am blessed to have chosen the path of immunization rather than addiction, and I am even more blessed to have been able to make the choice for myself. If there is a connection between allergy and addiction, I am confident that modern science will someday find the answer. It is an enormous puzzle well worth solving.

ADD AND ADHD
#attentiondeficitdisorderandattentiondeficithyperactivitydisorder-aredifficulttodiagnose

Even though I have never been diagnosed with Attention Deficit or Attention Deficit Hyperactivity Disorder, I sympathize with those who have. My allergy symptoms and those attributed to these conditions can often, on the surface, appear to be very similar. These chronic conditions include such general symptoms as attention difficulty, impulsiveness, and hyperactivity.

As a Montessori teacher in the early 1990's, we were trained to look for behavior and other signs related to ADD and ADHD in children. Aggressive behavior, lack of concentration, shifting back and forth between subjects or activities, center-of-attention syndrome, obsessive-compulsive tendencies, incomplete tasks, impulsive outbursts, resistance to routines, the need for frequent reminders, and so forth, were easy to recognize in the quiet, orderly classroom.

One of our students, a young four year-old boy, had a hard time sitting still. He was very intelligent, and very social. He enjoyed randomly calling out students' names to get their attention. He was disruptive, but in a playful way, and he responded well to reminders. We were working on helping him to respect boundaries, and we were also monitoring his congestion and other symptoms of allergy. The process was slow, and his parents, although cooperative, were impatient. They wanted us to "fix him" right away. We couldn't do that, of course, so they turned to his pediatrician for medication. Once he became medicated, he preferred to just sit quietly in a chair and watch the other children. His allergy symptoms remained unchanged. His family moved away that year, but I have often wondered what the prognosis would have been had they consulted an allergist as well. His was only one of many examples I encountered through the years.

As a rule, the children whose families chose to explore the allergy factor and make changes in their environments achieved significant progress but the process was more gradual. Significantly, their personalities and enthusiasm remained intact.

We have all seen crying, distressed children acting out in public. Criticizing the parents for not controlling them is easy to do. However, there is a chance that, like me, they are sensitive to ingredients in the public environment which makes it difficult for them to control their behavior, even if they want to. Allergens can manifest themselves into so many different behavioral reactions. As I have pointed out so many times before, human beings can be allergic even if they hardly ever sneeze. If I had a hyperactive, low-energy, unpredictable, or troubled child, I would want to explore all my options. If something as simple as a teacher's perfume unknowingly causes a child to be labeled and thus put on a possible lifetime regimen of strong medication, we as a society are not doing our job.

Of course I understand that my limited experience with a few children does not represent significant data. I simply provide these examples as food for thought about the holistic possibilities. I can't help but be concerned for the millions of children who have been diagnosed with ADD and/or ADHD and, without a voice of their own, are being unnecessarily medicated.

Allergy, ADD, and ADHD are not one and the same, but in my mind, looking back at all my years of complicated experiences, the similarities between them cannot be denied. There are so many intermingling signs and symptoms which could easily lead to an inaccurate diagnosis if we are too quick to assign a label. Even when a true attention deficit or hyperactivity disorder is determined, recognizing an accompanying allergic condition and treating it as well, could most surely be helpful in its management.

Adults, as well as children, can suffer from ADD and ADHD. While a diagnosis of adult onset can occur, many believe they have suffered from this condition since childhood. We are blessed these days with much more information and understanding among both the medical community and the general public. I know several adults, including extended family members, who have finally received an accurate ADHD diagnosis. For years, I have been encouraging them to be tested and treated for allergy, but to no avail. Their medication is truly helpful, but I wish they could know what it feels like to be allergy-free as well.

I have heard people joke about having imaginary ADD when they have trouble staying on task or when they are easily distracted by such things as seeing a squirrel out the window. Randomly yelling, "squirrel" may lighten the moment, and I understand the levity. However, to those who are truly suffering, and possibly covering up their problems by living in the shadows, it is far from a laughing matter.

I am encouraged by the fact that ongoing research is providing better insights into the treatments for ADD and ADHD. Hopefully, my observations and experiences have helped raise awareness as to the possible allergy connection when a diagnosis is being considered.

Discovering the Mother Hormone
#dehydroepiandrosteronedeficiencyisnotdesirable

DHEA is a steroidal hormone produced in the adrenal cortex, gonads, and brain. It is often called the "mother of all hormones" because it is more prolific than any other hormone produced by the adrenal glands. It is a powerful immune system booster. Like many of you, I had never heard of it. When Dr. Pienkowski discovered that my body was not producing it, I was curious.

When he explained that it was emerging as having therapeutic effects in medical conditions such as cardiovascular disease, diabetes, hypercholesterolemia (high levels of cholesterol in the blood), obesity, cancer, Alzheimer's disease, immune disorders, chronic fatigue and osteoporosis, my jaw dropped. I was at risk.

Symptoms of DHEA deficiency include persistent fatigue, anxiety, hypersensitivity to noise, loss of libido, dry eyes and skin, depression, and loss of hair.

The body's production of DHEA reaches a peak in the mid-twenties and declines progressively from then on. By the time you are in your seventies, the DHEA levels are only ten percent of what they were, but they are still present and they are important. Blood levels of DHEA apparently serve as a marker for many degenerative diseases and I feel fortunate that my levels are being tracked.

Studies at the National Institute of Mental Health in Bethesda, Maryland,[18] have shown that low blood levels of DHEA can better predict a heart attack than can high levels of cholesterol. Also, low levels of DHEA indicate increased risk of breast cancer more than any other marker. DHEA has also been associated with anti-aging properties and a general sense of well-being. Perhaps it contributes to my current healthy optimistic outlook and my ongoing "joie de vivre" which in my allergic past were conspicuously absent along with my nonexistent DHEA.

Dr. Pienkowski's discovery is amazing. We have no idea how long my body has not produced DHEA, and that will remain a mystery. Standard blood tests do not include DHEA evaluation. The good news is that he knows just what to do to restore my proper levels. A safe, effective, inexpensive supplement is available over the counter. It is a small white pill with no colorings or coatings to cause me trouble. I take 25 milligrams twice a day and ever since my diagnosis, my readings have been normal.

Few people would consider going to an allergist for routine blood work, but I am so glad I did. It may not have actually saved my life, but I am confident that restoring my DHEA levels has helped save my quality of life. Since there is a history of dementia and Alzheimer's in my family, perhaps I have dodged a bullet. It is important to note that I am not promoting DHEA as an additional supplement. That should be between you and your personal physician. I am just glad that my deficiency was discovered at an early age.

Several years ago, when I went for my yearly physical, I requested that DHEA be included in my bloodwork. My request was denied because "that is an allergist's matter." I was shocked, and I wondered if

---

18   www.nimh.nih.gov

insurance coverage was involved in that decision. No clear answer was provided other than the statement that "It is not in the mainstream." Apparently, DHEA deficiency can happen to anyone, and I was curious what allergy had to do with the fact that my body was no longer producing that important hormone. One would think that a general practitioner would be concerned to discover an irregularity of this sort. Apparently it was not an issue so it was necessary for me to repeat the process and schedule a second blood test at Dr. Pienkowski's office. To me, this duplication seemed expensive, repetitive, inconvenient, and unnecessary on many levels, but it was well worth it, nonetheless.

When I arrived for the second test at Dr. P.'s office, I asked the nurse if she understood why my insurance had to pay for two blood tests. She surmised that a specialist's evaluation was necessary because even if the general practitioner received the information, she "wouldn't know what to do with it." I wondered why they couldn't just share the results, but I didn't ask.

Fortunately, the DHEA connection to wellness is becoming more mainstream in the medical community. Just recently, Jennifer's physician suggested that, at age 45, she would benefit from taking a low-dose DHEA supplement. Hopefully, current DHEA research will continue to thrive, helping more and more people to solve their mysteries and benefit from the results.

Stolen Days and Unfinished Tasks

#allergensturnmorningmotivationintoafternoonfrustrationandeven-eningsedation

I am by nature a goal-oriented, organized and efficient person. I believe that projects once begun should be completed. It's a matter of respect. My children have heard me say on numerous occasions, "A job worth doing is worth doing well." Honoring commitments, either to myself or to others was always my intention. Allergy had other ideas.

Through the years, there were dishes left undone, letters half-written and never mailed, phone calls avoided and never returned, recipes untried, invitations not accepted, books checked out but never read, weddings and funerals not attended, television shows and movies watched but not remembered, friendships not developed, and thoughtful gifts intended, yet never baked or bought.

If you, the reader, were ever personally involved with any of the above, please understand that it was never about you. I would have done things differently if only I had had the ability to follow my heart.

My purpose in writing this section is to point out how easily allergy can affect behavior. If someone has a serious disability or disease, unfinished tasks and unachievable goals are readily accepted as part of the illness. In my experience, allergy was not considered a disease because its effects on the whole body, both mentally and physically, were not generally understood. Therefore, I was struggling on my own, trying to understand and reconcile my inabilities, and making excuses why things were left undone. My barrier was never about motivation or intent; it was about ability in the moment. As if I were out in the ocean, caught in a riptide, and constantly swimming for shore.

There were times when something as simple as sweeping the kitchen floor presented itself as a monumental task. I could drop something on the floor and say to myself, "That's okay, I'll pick it up later." Unless you have walked in my shoes, how could you understand something as trivial as not having the energy to lean down and pick up an object, even if it was nothing more than a crumpled up napkin. Scarlet O'Hara was famous for putting things off. There were times when monsters denied me the choice.

Everywhere I looked, I was reminded of something that needed to be done, and more often than not, I was the one who should be doing it. Obstacles kept blocking my path and almost every little thing took longer than it should have. Even when I heard the words, "Job well done," in my mind it was never enough. Autumn leaves remained in piles for someone else (Michael) to pick up. Trays of annual flowers enthusiastically bought in the spring often died before they were planted. Even if planted, regular watering was a challenge, and they died on the vine. Killing plants and flowers was difficult to accept, especially for a florist. Had the responsibility been left to me, the grass would have probably been three feet high and the cars would have fallen apart in the driveway.

Piles of unwashed and unfolded laundry are not uncommon for many families, but for me those mounting stacks became a symbol of the things I left incomplete. Now I know that in addition to the scented items, even such a minor task as cleaning lint from the dryer vent made me feel light-headed. I avoided that chore as long as I could. Years later, when I discovered dryer balls, fabric softener became obsolete. Whoever invented these plastic balls deserves a medal.

Sometimes I either forgot or didn't get back to the washer in time and the clothes soured. Their allergic effect on me was the same as mildew. Since my sense of smell was diminished from the allergy, sometimes I wouldn't be aware that the shirt I was wearing had actually soured before going into the dryer. Mildew monsters were then able to follow me around until I finally realized what was happening. At that point the cycle began again and that entire load had to be identified and washed all over again. For years, I felt caught up in a whirlpool of lost days and never-ending incompletions.

I was concerned that I might be sending mixed messages to the children. I did not want to be one of those parents who said, "Do as I say and not as I do." I wanted them to always be responsible, complete their assignments on time, and follow through with all their chores. I worried that they might feel I was expecting things of them that I did not expect of myself. I did not want to come across as a hypocrite. Family meetings and good conversation helped them to understand. Were it not for Michael's support, my guilt could have gotten out of hand. We prioritized, and only I know what experiences we could have had if we had known then what we know now. Thankfully, both Andy and Jennifer have become successful, responsible adults and they barely remember the days of turmoil. All is well.

One time during the flower shop years, my mother told me that my grandmother was bringing some family members up from

Cleveland to visit. I panicked. What was I to do? I loved them so, but our house was a mess. What would they think of me? There was no time to clean and tidy up properly, even if I had the ability to do so. I felt helpless and I was an emotional wreck. I worried that they might be disappointed in me, thinking I had let my values down. Michael was willing to help, but at that point, I couldn't even think clearly enough to give him a list. Everything was just one big blur.

Mother finally convinced me that they were coming to visit the family and me, because they loved us. They were not coming to check on the status of my housekeeping, and they would never judge. I finally gave in. When the guests arrived, after hugs and greetings all around, something changed. They saw that we needed help and they began to pitch in. A healthy person most likely would have appreciated the well-intentioned help, but I was horrified. I felt embarrassed and betrayed. In my mind, it was about the housecleaning, after all. The emotional stress I experienced that day stayed with me for a very long time. Now we know that I was the one, not the house, in need of help. A non-allergified Tollie would have handled the situation differently. My monsters not only left me with unfinished tasks, but they distorted my perception as well.

For a long time after that day, I made every possible excuse to avoid having company. My allergy and its powers of interruption caused us to become more and more socially isolated. I began to hide.

Michael never complained about the unfinished nature of our lives, as if he had a sixth sense that something beyond our comprehension was going on. He must have been more frustrated than he let on, but he never blamed me for anything. He compared me to a lovely garden spider, constantly trying to spin her perfect web. I couldn't see it that way, and I didn't really take it as a compliment. I just wanted to be normal.

I am creative and artistic by nature. Many of my crafts, artwork, and decorating projects were left incomplete or at best I took a really long time getting back to them. Paint brushes were left unclean and had to be thrown away. Styles changed and by the time I revisited them, many projects were no longer in vogue. Perhaps I love antiques because rather than losing their appeal, they just get "antiquier." Some of my best intentions remain unfinished still today. I have learned to stick with water colors, acrylics, and non-oil-based products these days and the artist in me is flourishing. I have started painting a mural on our patio wall. It is incomplete because I am so busy, but I have finally discovered the value of proudly calling an unfinished project my "work in progress." Michael calls me his "Salvadore Tollie," and we laugh.

My life changed dramatically when Dr. Pienkowski came to the rescue. With his help, I was able to arrive at the indisputable conclusion that my frustrating experiences, previously deemed inexplicable, had an explanation after all. The relief I felt when I was finally able to hold my allergies responsible for placing these obstacles in my path is indescribable. Little by little, as I got into my treatment, tasks began to reach completion. The process was slow, but confidence in my abilities was no longer eroding and we were finally getting back on track. I have heard it said that the path to success is paved with good intentions. Wouldn't it be amazing if the world finally realized that allergy monsters could be responsible for providing some of the roadblocks.

Chasing Numbers on the Scale
OBESITY

#celebrateyoursizebutstaywithinsafemarginsforyourhealth

Throughout my life I have had problems maintaining my weight. Not major problems in the early years, but ups and downs. I have watched weight come and energy go. At my wedding in 1968, I weighed 106 pounds, less than I weighed in the third grade. The highest number I have seen is 245. My climb into obesity was a rocky and complicated road. Little did I know back then, but it too was allergy-related.

For those of us who struggle to keep our weight within healthy limits, finding a plan that really works is a monumental task. Temptation lurks around every corner, and there is no "one size fits all" solution, as far as I can tell. We live in a superficial society, often plagued with unrealistic expectations. Even the word obese can be perceived as hurtful when applied to those of us who are trying our hardest to succeed. Along my allergic journey, I received more compliments when I lost a few pounds than when, for example, my constant coughing subsided or I lost the dark circles under my eyes.

Before I realized that allergies were interfering with my weight loss efforts, I was constantly searching for answers. Not excuses, but answers. Looking at pictures of my ancestors (and there are many), I see mostly slender figures, both men and women, so I have ruled out genetics as a major factor. Great-grandmother Moore, on my dad's side, was described in her day as "pleasantly plump." As a young girl, I thought that hugging her was like hugging a giant marshmallow. There was always a large glass canister of homemade sugar cookies on her kitchen counter and we were allowed to help ourselves without asking. If overweight issues are genetic, the condition apparently skipped a couple of generations and landed on me.

I was fairly slender when Michael and I began our career in the floral industry in the late 1970's. Within a short time, I began to gain weight. Hazel Price, the kind and gentle soft-spoken shop owner, said to me one morning, "You look puffy." She was right, of course, but at the time it hurt my feelings. Before I knew what was happening, I had gained 20 pounds. We blamed it on the fast food restaurant across the street, grabbing pastries from a box on hectic mornings, and dinner on the go. Michael and the children were not gaining weight, and perhaps that should have been a clue, but I was yet to recognize my allergic constitution, much less its contribution to the piling on of pounds. Looking back, I recognize it now.

Weight Watchers was big in those days and I signed up with great expectations. Their program was basically about portion control. Few processed foods were allowed but I do remember the artificial low-fat margarine. The plan was nutritious (we had to eat liver every week and lots of fish) and within a few weeks I lost 16 pounds. The strict routine proved to be too demanding, and soon I was back to the old ways of trying to manage my health, my family, and my career. I barely had time to notice as the pounds came creeping back.

Through the following years, I tried various "diets" which seemed to work for others, but not for me. Measuring and counting calories was time-consuming and difficult to manage during my allergified years. Convenience foods soon crept back into the kitchen.

I tried various "helpful hints" such as small plates, one meal per day, six meals per day, chopsticks, chewing each bite 20 times, and so forth. None of these gimmicks helped at all.

One doctor explained that my extra pounds and my chronic energy deficit were related to metabolism. He suggested that I should have a small snack every two or three hours every day. His idea was not helpful. If food energizes you, the plan could make sense. It had the opposite effect on me. Now we know that I was simply re-introducing the food allergens which made me sleepy in the first place.

At one point, Michael and I decided to try the popular Atkins diet. Michael didn't need to lose much, and the program worked quickly for him. Even when I was eating only lettuce, celery, tuna, and some sort of artificially sweetened powdered drink mix, the scale would not budge. I could not reach ketosis, and I finally gave up.

The following summer, Michael's sister Penny came to visit. We three decided to try the new Weight Watchers program together. Pumpkin muffins and zucchini cookies with artificially sweetened cream cheese, diet gelatin, diet sodas, and diet bread, along with lo-fat everything were the norm. Michael lost a few pounds, even though he drifted from the program at times. After three months, Penny lost 28 pounds. I lost three. Naturally, I was distraught, but more than anything, I was determined. Detective DeGraw set out on a mission. Whoever these monsters were, I was not going to let them win.

The one encouraging motivation which has constantly accompanied my struggles with obesity is Michael's support. Never once has he said anything disparaging about my weight. Still today, my eyes rim with tears, just thinking about how fortunate I am to have this gentle giant in my life.

At various weight-loss meetings, I heard other women complain about their low self-esteem, and how they were shamed and criticized by husbands with unrealistic expectations about their figures. They were accused of "letting themselves go," even though they were trying their hardest to lose weight. I felt sorry for the lady who stopped for fast food on the way home to cook dinner, disposing of the evidence in someone else's trash can, and the man who kept snacks and a cooler hidden in the trunk of his car. Their stories were not mine, and I never needed food to replace affection because I had plenty of the real thing. However, I do empathize with those who feel uncomfortable, wondering if they are being judged by others, based on their size. I always hoped that if I could find my own answers, it would help them as well.

I began reading every weight-loss article I could get my hands on. Well-intentioned words just didn't ring true to me. My midsection continued to expand. There is a huge difference between a hard and a jiggly abdomen. I had them both. One front-page magazine article addressed the problem of abdominal bloating. The author's intention was to provide a solution for the growing number of obese potbellied Americans. I was optimistic, hoping for a medical breakthrough. I was disappointed, once again. The main culprits, the story maintained, were chewing gum, gulping foods, drinking while eating, and not sitting up straight. Taking a walk after meals would help, as well as exchanging white flour for celery, unsweetened cranberry juice, and grapefruit. "If you have a beer belly," the author advised, "quit drinking beer."

Seriously? Not that some of this isn't good advice, but it convinced me for good that I had to find the answers by studying my own self. No one else was able to help me.

I have a theory about when Americans first began to get fat. Beginning in the mid-1950's, canned mushroom soup casseroles topped with American cheese and a thick layer of buttery Ritz crackers, along with salty creamed chipped beef on toast points were all the rage. Frozen TV dinners, advertised as healthy and nutritious, began to appear on our tables several times a week and we sat in front of the television to eat them on our newly purchased TV trays. Artificially flavored, empty-calorie or sugary soft drinks replaced freshly squeezed juices. Colorful super-sweet cereals replaced home-made oatmeal, corn flakes, and shredded wheat.

Bottled sweet mixers and flavored alcoholic beverages replaced a simple "scotch and soda," or something "on the rocks." Five o'clock cocktail hour included cheesy dips, Vienna sausages, flavored potato chips, assorted candy and canapes before dinner. And then along came home-delivered pizza and fast food. We were doomed. America became addicted to the luxurious, sweet, salty, delicious processed fake foods.

These dietary changes obviously opened a path to extra fats and calories, but I see an allergy factor as well. When all these multi-ingredient items hit our menus, our bodies were bombarded with more and more items to which we became allergic. Our bodies do not always interpret these lab-created chemicals as nutrition, and so our appetites likely increase and we remain hungry for real food. The problems are then passed on down through the generations.

The more I searched for solutions, the more discouraged I became. Finding possible contributors to my weight problems did nothing to help me eliminate them. As soon as I fit in one puzzle piece, another would fall out. A few of my findings actually did appear significant. I know now that allergy affects my taste buds and my sense of smell. I realized that a lot of my eating was out of habit, and I had no indicator telling me when to stop. My "hunger hormones" were doing a poor job of helping me to understand the difference between hunger and satiety. Cortisol is a steroidal hormone which regulates metabolism and immune response. Its levels rise with corticosteroid medication and stress. We now know that too much cortisol encompassing the body over time contributes to weight gain, especially around the midsection. I continued journaling, trying to make a connection between what I ate and how I felt. I couldn't gain control, but

I remained motivated. I was convinced that if there were fewer cells in my body producing IgE's, my allergies would become less able to encourage obesity. If I lost weight, my allergies would be less severe. I wanted to retrain my body, but I also had to retrain the monsters. It was a daunting task, much like the conundrum of which comes first, the chicken or the egg.

WHY WORKING OUT WASN'T WORKING
#irefusetobedefinedbynumbersonascale

Many people believe that working out is the best answer in any endeavor to lose weight. The healthy benefits of exercise are manifold and cannot be denied. In my allergic state, working out had an insignificant effect on the numbers on my scale, but the more physically active I became, the better I felt. I was rewarded far beyond my original expectations.

In the early stages of my treatment, I began to visualize myself as a physically fit person. At first it was only a dream, but the motivation was real. My energy was always highest on cool early mornings in the spring, but every walking routine was quickly interrupted by the seasonal pollen.

I was a fairly good golfer in my teenage years, so as I was recovering, that sport seemed to be an excellent choice. Walking the course was good exercise for the first few holes, but trudging up the fairway towards the ninth green while extremely allergified was pure misery. The theory back then was that taking salt tablets was the answer. Those large white tablets were anything but helpful to me.

Even moderate heat was unbearable (sun allergy) and I longed for the coolness of "The Nineteenth Hole." These days, if you are allergic, golf carts provide a welcome solution.

Backyard croquet, badminton, and whiffle ball with the children and grandchildren were just a few of the family activities which for me were a challenge. I was competing with my monsters much more than I was competing with them. I was better at serving lemonade from my indoor kitchen. Being allergic and overweight in an athletic family left me feeling "odd man out." I was proud to sit in the bleachers, cheering them on as "Number One Fan," but I always wondered how it would feel to actually compete.

At age 55, my weight was well over 200 pounds. At just over five feet tall, I was still not healthy, even though my treatable symptoms were inching toward remission. Those of you who are allergic and are able to get your immunizations at an earlier age will be blessed with many more active years to spend with your families, and the benefits will enrich your lives beyond measure.

So in my late fifties, I signed up for the "Weigh to Go" program at Ft. Sanders Health and Fitness Center in Knoxville. It was (and still is) a state-of-the-art facility. I hired a personal trainer who designed my food menus and graded my daily journals. The plan was expensive, but the monetary incentive was a driving force in my determination to succeed. I drove the forty miles three times a week, eating celery and pretzels on my way there and grapes and cheese on the way home. Now I know that considering my food allergies, eating the same foods every day was not the best idea.

I worked hard, both individually and with my group of about ten people. At first, there were good results. I lost a couple of pounds and my strength increased. Body fat, lean muscle mass, fat weight and waist circumference all improved, even though tests showed that oxygen was not effectively reaching my muscles. One man commented to my trainer, "I have never seen anyone work so hard and look so happy." For someone who, in the past could barely make it through a Richard Simmons video, I was encouraged.

Before long, however, those awful allergy monsters once again reared their ugly heads. Gradually, others in my group dropped out one by one, as they lost their weight and met their goals. After nearly seven months, I had lost a grand total of seven pounds. My trainer was baffled as to why this intense program was not working for me. The more we discussed and tried to analyze my dilemma, the more often she said to me, "You really ought to write a book." Of course I was healthier from my workout experience, but obesity still reigned supreme.

Since I had no other medical issues, I hold my allergies responsible for the mysteries surrounding my muscles. My family can verify how strictly I adhered to the program, and I did not cheat. Why the program worked so well for others and not for me, remains unknown. I know that floor exercises were difficult because I became light-headed and dizzy any time my face was near the carpets or the mats. The problem was chemical outgassing, I presume. Yoga and Pilates were impossible. The recommended food plan was not designed around my food allergies, because they were not yet clearly understood. Fragrances associated with other members could have played a part as well. Perhaps it was just the nature of my allergic constitution. At any rate, I finally realized that I could no longer justify the expenditure of time and money and so, reluctantly, I called it quits. I cried all the way home.

About a year later, I decided to try again. I joined a local fitness club, not far from home. I just wanted to see what I could do on my own. My hopes were high and my expectations were low. The following story will probably seem strange to most of you, but I remember how it felt to actually run for the first time in my adult life. It took courage. There was an indoor track which ran on an upper level around the perimeter of the building. One morning I was walking as usual when I suddenly realized I was alone on the track. I gathered my nerve, and decided to see what would happen if I started to run. I had no idea what to do with my arms and hands. I began, hesitatingly at first, to lift my feet off the floor, and before I knew it, I was running! I breathed deeply, and it felt like I was flying. "Just running" must seem like a simple thing to most people, but it was one of the most exhilarating times of my life. Tears streamed down my cheeks as I circled the track. I was experiencing a miracle.

My message to you, the reader, is a bit of a dichotomy. On the one hand, I see great value in good exercise. On the other hand, I hope you aren't discouraged if allergy gets in your way. My workout experiences, all wrapped up in my all-encompassing allergic constitution, represent the extreme. Had I been more knowledgeable ahead of time, perhaps the monsters and I could have danced to a different tune. Allergic people, even asthmatics, can work out successfully, and if you are among that population, I wish you well.

THE CANDIDA CONNECTION
#candidaalbicansovergrowthcreatedthebiggestmonsterofthemall

I was just about to decide, "Well, this is it. The last few missing puzzle pieces may just have to remain missing. I am out of new ideas, so it is time to accept life as it is and leave the rest for experts to discover for future generations." My monsters were kept at a distance, and I knew how to handle those rare occasions when they tried to invade my space. My family finally understood everything, and they had learned to aim their anger and frustration at the monsters instead of at me. The word "allergified" was practically missing from my vocabulary, and Dr. Pienkowski was only a phone call away. I could live with being overweight if necessary, as long as it wasn't causing other health issues. The pharmacy no longer kept any active prescriptions in my file, and that was a huge milestone. Food allergy is destined to be my lifelong partner, and I can accept that as well. It was time to move on, appreciate my accomplishments and look forward to what a healthy future had to offer.

There was still one nagging issue, a significant missing puzzle piece, which eluded me through the years and remained in my mind unconnected to allergy. Although I had no history of hives or the "heartbreak of psoriasis" as the commercial described it, I did have an intermittent rash on my lower abdomen just where the skin folds over. Outbreaks presented as an angry red and painful skin condition, much like prickly heat, a baby's diaper rash, or what some people refer to as jock itch.

Off and on through the years I sought help from my family physician and my dermatologist. There were no answers. Once in the early 1990's my family physician said, "Oh, that's what fat people get when skin rolls over and touches skin." It was an awkward moment I will never forget. I had not considered myself "fat," at that point and it hurt my feelings. He had no other solutions. The implication was, "lose weight or just deal with it." I was reluctant to bring the subject up again.

Several years later, when I began getting yearly skin checks, I asked my dermatologist if he could help. He prescribed a cream used for athlete's foot. It didn't help at all. A few years later another dermatologist suggested I shower often and keep the skin dry. A hair dryer might help. I could try an antiperspirant, but it would probably cause an itchy rash. Still no help, so I continued on my own. I tried baby powder, cornstarch, antiperspirants, diaper cream, zinc oxide and baking soda. Nothing worked. I never made the allergy connection as I dealt privately with the painful episodes throughout the years.

When I went for my annual allergy check-up in April of 2013, I just happened to be having a flare-up. For some reason, I suddenly thought to ask Dr. Pienkowski if he could offer any advice. After one quick glance, he said, "Candidiasis. You need steroid cream." Once again, magic words. He prescribed a specific corticosteroid and anti-fungal ointment. After using it properly for two full weeks, this painful condition I had put up with for all those years was completely cured. Now whenever I feel the slightest tingle as an indicator of a possible recurrence, I simply apply a tiny amount for a couple of days and the painful rash never develops.

To point out how misunderstood this condition often is, I once asked a dermatologist if he would write a refill prescription for my cream. He said no, because too much of it would cause stretch marks. I was astounded. First of all, I would not use "too much." Why did he assume people are not smart enough to follow directions? And second, why would I be concerned about a few cosmetic stretch marks if it meant this intolerable painful condition could disappear? It was puzzling, and I went home without my prescription. Back to Dr. P.

As important as this diagnosis was, something monumental was about to happen. The word "Candidiasis" was destined to change my life. I rushed home to my computer and began my research. Almost immediately I met Candida Albicans, the biggest monster of them all.

There was a clear connection to the remaining mysteries in my life, specifically my obesity. Puzzle pieces which had remained missing since childhood began flying into place. Those flying puzzle pieces made me very, very happy.

Candida Albicans is a fungus (a form of yeast) which causes a condition in the body known as Candida Related Complex (CRC). Candida yeast occurs naturally in the human body. It is necessary for optimal health, but when its population grows out of control, it can weaken the immune system, affect digestion, encourage weight gain and damage the intestinal wall, allowing toxic by-products to enter the bloodstream. The more I read, the more I became convinced that my Candidiasis was more than just a rash. In addition to abnormal weight gain, other significant symptoms associated with this condition include joint pain, chronic fatigue, food allergy, brain fog, anxiety, sinus issues, vaginal yeast infections, thrush (a white coating on the tongue), urinary tract infections, scalp problems, athlete's foot, premenstrual syndrome (PMS), emotional disturbance, cravings for sweets, stress, chemical sensitivity, and depression.

As is common with these often misunderstood conditions, I encountered countless opinions as to the role Candidiasis plays in health-related issues. Surely the similarity between these symptoms associated with Candidiasis and those associated with allergy are more than a mere coincidence. My goal here is to alert you, the reader, to the possibility that in addition to allergy, an overgrowth of Candida Albicans could be complicating your search for medical answers. Of course we all react in different ways, and as always, I had to be my own lead detective. Even though it took me a while, I was finally able to connect the dots.

Even though there is no definitive test available to doctors, there is a procedure called the "spit test" which some claim to be a reliable indicator of an overgrowth of yeast in the body. It is not scientifically proven, but it appears to be an accurate indicator of problems and progress in my situation. If you are curious, you can find the instructions on the internet. As with anything you find online, you should evaluate its significance for yourself.

CRC is in the early stages of being recognized in the medical community. Because the symptoms overlap and are so complex, Candida overgrowth is often undiagnosed, misdiagnosed, or ignored altogether. The same appears to be true with many allergic conditions. Cures cannot be consistently predicted and in the field of medicine, this creates a problem. There are times when I just feel like saying, "Welcome to my world!"

As I discovered the possible contributors to my Candida overgrowth, there was not a doubt in my mind. I was a victim and I probably had been for most, if not all, of my life. When I first heard of the Candida connection to scalp problems, I was even more convinced. Various research conducted during the last 20 years substantiates the theory that dandruff and other scalp conditions are medical in nature, not cosmetic. Scientists now believe that an overgrowth of a microorganism called malassezia, (a yeast-like fungus) and Candida play a major role in causing itchy, scaly scalp and dandruff. Allergy to hair products, food allergy and other dietary conditions such as nutritional deficiencies can also play a part. As skin cells die and fall off, they appear as the white flakes we see in our hair and on our clothing.

If the amount of commercials I see on television is an indicator, a large segment of Americans suffer from dandruff-related problems. Unfortunately, many people still believe that dandruff is caused by dry scalp, frequent shampooing and poor hygiene. They are self-conscious and because so many consider it a cosmetic rather than a medical issue, it is often not reported. This of course impedes the urgency and progress of Candida-related medical research.

Restoring the pH balance on the scalp can help relieve the discomfort. There are medications available, but if you are interested in trying a home remedy, products like coconut oil, lemon juice and apple cider vinegar can be very effective scalp treatments. My discovery of Nioxin and Bosley products, as previously mentioned, helps me immensely, and I use these products for body wash as well. This limits my exposure to additional chemicals, natural ingredients and fragrances, to which I am potentially allergic. If only we had known in my childhood what we understand now. After considering my lifetime of at least twice yearly antibiotics, adrenal dysfunction, prolonged stress, a mouthful of mercury fillings, years of taking oral contraceptives, chlorinated pools, fluoridated water, immune system deficiency, multiple allergies, and a diet which I thought to be healthy but was actually feeding my Candida, I soon realized I was a prime target. Even newborn babies are susceptible if nursing mothers are taking antibiotics. It could be possible that I have had this overgrowth since infancy.

My first plan of action was to begin the Candida elimination diet. I learned to identify foods which feed the Candida and foods which starve it. The plan is simple and nutritious, emphasizing such things as meat, fish, eggs, vegetables, nuts, seeds, yogurt, natural oils, herbs, and spices. Fruits, dairy, and other carbohydrates are incorporated gradually as your body learns to tolerate them. I looked forward to shrinking my swollen abdomen, which was reported to be one of the first signs of success linked to reducing Candida overload. I don't like the term "belly bloat," even though we hear it all the time. Probably because my mother would tell me, "cows have bellies and people have stomachs." Regardless of what you call it, my swollen abdomen was a constant reminder of my obesity, and I really wanted it to go away. I was cautiously optimistic.

As soon as I began the Candida diet, amazing things began to happen. I avoided all the expensive supplements, instant cleanses, and guaranteed cures promoted on most of the associated websites. I wanted to do it my own way. My detective skills were never more important than in this endeavor.

My newfound food program was easy to follow and not overly restrictive. I never felt deprived, as there were no portion limits as long as a food was not on the forbidden list. I was amazed at how well I felt as I began limiting or eliminating artificial sweeteners, refined sugars, flour and various carbohydrates. I discovered many new recipes and delicious foods I had never even tasted before. Soon Michael wanted to "have what you're having." Within a short time, he lost 30 pounds. I strongly advise anyone with a weight problem to consider giving this food plan a try, even for a short period of time.

It is said that over half of the antibiotics in this country are sold to the livestock industry, which means that they are in our meat, eggs, and dairy products as well. The stimulating growth hormones which fatten up our pigs and cattle might also be fattening us up as consumers. We are all mammals, after all! The average person has little control over this growing problem, but if you determine you have a Candida overgrowth, unknowingly adding antibiotics to your diet could very well interfere with your progress.

If you are fortunate enough to have access to grass fed beef, it is healthy and anti-inflammatory, and it does not feed Candida. I discovered the amazing sweetening power of pure stevia, so I can still feed my sweet tooth without feeding the yeast as well. Daily servings of full fat plain yogurt provide probiotics (good bacteria) which crowd out the Candida and help restore the proper pH levels to the digestive tract. We like it better than sour cream. I also discovered the delicious wonders of coconut oil, which contains caprylic acid, an anti-microbial known to kill yeasts like Candida, either by ingestion or topical application. If I could, I would bathe in it! I learned that commercially produced flavor enhancers such as MSG and others are nucleic acids, derived from yeast. They are associated with increased food cravings, so I avoid them when I can identify them, but they hide among other ingredients. You can find a basic Candida elimination diet on the internet, but beware of sites which are hawking their elixirs, cleanses, and tonics. As always, you should first consult a doctor before embarking on a new program.

Along with food lists, I also learned the importance of taking small bites and chewing food thoroughly. The longer food sits in your stomach, the more chance it has to ferment and turn to sugar, which feeds the Candida. Yeast attaches to vegetables and moves more rapidly through the stomach as well, so our mothers were on to something when they taught us to eat lots of vegetables, eat them slowly, and chew them well!

As soon as I began to put my new food plan into practice, the pounds began falling off. Within six months I was seventy pounds lighter and my constant "watermelon abdomen" was a thing of the past. I have not regained those lost pounds, but I still have to be careful with my food choices. If I get careless or eat too much sugar and processed foods, my cravings return and I begin to feel more swollen and less energetic. My weight always fluctuates, even within ten or twenty pounds, but after all I have been through, it is an easy dilemma to accept. Most of all, the ability to control my Candidiasis is a blessing and I am forever grateful to Dr. Pienkowski for his accurate diagnosis.

My lifelong condition was, and in some ways still is, extreme. Yours may be equally important but less complicated. Those of us with severe food allergy may never completely conquer Candida, but we can keep it at bay. Wherever you fall in the spectrum, Candida Albicans may be interfering in your search for the healthy, happy, human condition. Foods which are good for food allergies are not necessarily Candida friendly, and vice versa. For example, it is good to eat anti-inflammatory and anti-Candida foods on a daily basis, but five-day rotations are better for food allergy. Well-cooked foods are best for allergies, but raw vegetables are more helpful in fighting Candida. So far, I have found the balance which seems to be working for me. As a slimmer, healthier, happier person, I am invigorated. I anticipate the future with a youthful outlook, and I doubt the term elderly will ever apply.

Public Perception and Raising Awareness
TELEVISION AND ADVERTISING
#thepowerofthecyclopscannotbedenied

Television sets are present in nearly every home in America. Even those without computers have access to programs on TV. Therein lies a tremendous ability to influence the attitudes and opinions of the everyday consumer. Sometimes the influence is healthy, but sometimes it is distorted. I rarely see instances in which the plight of allergic individuals is accurately portrayed.

Commercials about allergy medications are frustrating. Sneezing, sniffling, wheezing, coughing, and so forth are portrayed as the most miserable symptoms on the face of the Earth. Beginning every spring, these products proclaim to be the cure-all and end-all to every allergy-sufferer's misery. The cycle begins again when autumn arrives. Of course allergies are serious business. That is why I am writing this book. Popping a pill or two every few hours or spraying the nose with possibly addicting over-the-counter nasal sprays over and over again is not the only answer. I am concerned for the segment of our population who can barely afford these medicines, and who therefore suffer in silence. I have yet to see a mention of immunization as an alternative. Advertisers are counting on all this repeat business, but I am reminded of Einstein's theory of insanity. Treating the same symptoms over and over again, year after year, and expecting a different result is only wishful thinking at best.

I wish someone would create a television show about an allergic family. It could be funny and really entertaining, as well as informative and consciousness-raising. It won't happen, of course, because if any form of successful immunization were involved, finding sponsors might prove impossible. More public awareness would interfere with sales of their advertised products.

Television programs with allergy components have always caught my attention. For example, there was a talk show about a newlywed couple who had a cat problem. He hates her cats and she has loved them for six years. They love each other but he is mean to the cats. The host's observation was that the husband should be able to control his behavior unless he had some "weird cat neurosis." Disrespecting the cats was paramount to disrespecting his wife. The man had dark circles under his eyes which looked to me like allergic shiners, and he was clearly in a state of lethargy and frustration. Instead of receiving helpful advice, he was being criticized and chastised. Apparently, suggesting an allergy evaluation was out of the realm of reason, but that alternative seemed perfectly logical to me.

Another memorable show dealt with the subject of "open mouth syndrome." Rather than recognizing a possible medical issue, the host jokingly showed a picture of a young man with a blank expression on his face. His jaw dropped, his mouth hung open, and they called him "The Village Idiot." The show also associated the open mouth syndrome with obese children, as if they did not have sense enough to close their mouths. These analogies seemed cruel to me. Breathing through a stopped-up nose is impossible, and it has nothing to do with intelligence. These victims need to be treated for their conditions, and their disparagers need sensitivity training, in my humble opinion.

Watching professional baseball, especially in the spring, we see players running the bases with their mouths open. One of our favorite players has dark circles under his eyes. He misses games, suffering from "flu-like symptoms." He is clearly allergic, and the same scenario repeats itself year after year. He is not alone, yet for some reason, athletes are reluctant to hold their allergies responsible, as if acknowledging them is admitting to some sort of weakness. If I were a coach, I would encourage all my players to be tested for allergies, just in case. If treatments were indicated, they could begin in the off-season and all the unwanted symptoms could diminish by the time spring training rolled around. Allergy awareness could become a secret weapon, and just like individual nutrition and conditioning, it could give the team a real edge.

On a positive note, a judge in Virginia was being credited with rescuing many marriages from divorce. He was a man ahead of his time. He refused to grant a divorce until both parties were tested for allergies. The documentary referenced an engaged couple struggling to save their relationship. He was convinced she disliked his family because she became uncomfortable and irritable whenever they spent time in his parents' home. She insisted she liked them very well. Their dispute was resolved when the couple realized she was allergic to the gas heat, appliances, and fireplace in the family home. The wedding proceeded as planned.

Not long ago, I came across a popular sitcom which depicted a father counselling his ten-year-old child who was being teased at school. He asks how things are going and the child replies that all is well because the bully is allergic to peanuts. "I can take him out with a handful of trail mix," the child replies, and the audience erupts into raucous laughter. I guess it was amusing on the surface, but it was disturbing as well. Something as serious has a life-threatening peanut allergy should not be taken so lightly. We can do better.

One last example concerns hypochondria. The host was laughing about a guest who constantly missed work and couldn't keep a job. He made fun of her "crazy excuses" and her outlandish insistence that she suffered from "unexplained, uneasy, achy feelings" that could not be confirmed by her doctor as an actual disease. The way he insinuated she was making her story up to get attention was heartbreaking to me. I was reminded of my own mysterious symptoms which defied explanation for such a long time. In the end, they labeled her a "hypochondriac," and she cried.

Members of the media have an opportunity to make huge contributions to the overall health of our nation by unveiling new ways of looking at previously vague conceptions and misconceptions regarding medical mysteries. Allergy is a welcome possible explanation to the previously unexplainable. Education can make a huge difference in society and it can provide an even greater impact when confusion becomes grounded by surrounding it with facts.

THE WIMPY KID
#debunkingthewimpykidanddethroningallergybullies

One of my goals in writing this book is to dispel the image of the "wimpy kid." You know, the one in glasses with the red nose who is a little bit chubby, not athletic, labeled lazy, always out of breath, constantly sneezing and reaching for tissues, gazing out the window instead of paying attention in class. The individual perceived as an open-mouthed idiot who is actually a really nice person.

I myself don't fit this stereotype, but I empathize and sympathize with those who do. For years the media has portrayed these children as the sissies, the wimpy kids, the ones with twitchy, wrinkly rabbit noses. To me they are clearly allergic. Making fun of them is unkind, and they should be placed in the same classification as anyone else with an illness or a disability. As I became healthier, I was able to expand my focus and broaden my horizons beyond my own personal microcosm. The bigger picture alerted me to the disturbing realization that many parents, teachers, siblings and peers were caught up in this hurtful stereotype. They trivialized significant, often debilitating events and subjected the innocent to ridicule.

Why do people make fun of allergy? So many people want to avoid admitting they are allergic, as if it is some sort of character deficiency. They try to come up with every imaginable excuse. It's just a cold. I didn't sleep well, so my eyes are red. The dark circles are from being tired and a lack of sleep. Cucumber slices, eye cream and concealer will help. It's just a morning cough, or a smoker's cough. I've picked up a virus. Just a little indigestion. Something I ate. And on and on.

When my treatment began to help me relate my long list of symptoms to the allergic condition, friends and family still tried to convince me that these unusual reactions were caused by something else. They were tired of hearing about allergies. "Allergy simply cannot be the answer to everything," they said. With all due respect to my loved ones, they were wrong. No one ever came up with another answer or explanation and the allergy diagnosis prevails.

I have spent many, many years defending unkind imaging and trying to convince others of the far-reaching unusual connections to allergy. It has truly been an uphill battle, but one I am intent on winning. The hardest concept for others to grasp is that holding my allergies responsible is not an excuse for anything. It is an explanation. How can an allergic reaction cause you to be angry? Or lethargic? Or sad? Something else must be going on. My own mother, who admitted to a lifelong cat allergy, was sympathetic to the itching and sniffles but could not accept the fact that a cat could cause a headache.

I sympathize with the image of the wimpy kid. I am here in his or her defense. It is completely unfair to believe that these allergic reactions and behaviors can simply be corrected at will. If you are a wimpy kid, or if you know one, I am here to tell you that there are answers. Admitting to far-reaching and unusual allergic symptoms, seeking the proper treatment and sharing information can go a long way towards erasing this negative image. One of my goals is to enlighten the deniers and the skeptics who are indulging in preconceptions and misconceptions by providing them with truthful awareness.

I have just recently encountered the term "allergy bullying." It is a horrifying concept. According to FARE (Food Allergy Research and Education)[19], one third of children with food allergies report being bullied at school. Six million American children suffer from food allergy, and for some of them, a severe reaction can occur just by touching a certain food or by inhaling airborne particles from opening a bag. Allergic children face a huge challenge when trying to eat safely away from home while enduring the threat of being ostracized or bullied by his or her peers. Many live in fear each day, knowing that ingesting a certain food could cause them to stop breathing.

For some reason, the stigma associated with allergies is escalating among our young population. Children are being harassed and tormented by the threat of peanut butter smeared on their faces or peanuts hidden in their food. Offending food is being thrown at them and bullies threaten to make them eat something against their will. Raising awareness is crucial if we are to protect these children. Allergies are not a laughing matter. The possibility is hard to imagine, but from a legal standpoint, if one child forced another to eat a peanut, and the child died from anaphylaxis, would it be murder? I pray we never have to find out. We must educate our population, and especially our children, about the seriousness of these issues. Understanding increases compassion, and compassion is a very good thing.

---

19   www.foodallergy.org

SEARCHING FOR THE CURE

bigpharmaneedstogetonboardbutdollarsholdthemback

Before reaching the conclusion of my (previously) allergic life history, I would be remiss if I didn't address the subject of finding a cure. Scientists all around the world, including here in East Tennessee, are working valiantly on behalf of allergy sufferers. The medical community still knows little about how allergies actually work, largely because we all react so differently. Due to the complexity of allergic disease, its influence is not yet clearly understood, but answers are beginning to appear along the horizon. Dr. Pienkowski is involved in significant peanut allergy research, and he is now even able to desensitize for milk. I pray we are on the verge of a cure.

Although those involved in medical research are making steady progress toward developing either a preventative vaccine or an actual cure, lack of funding and lack of incentive on the part of the large pharmaceutical companies, insurance agencies, various governmental regulatory agencies, and others continue to stand in the way. As you evaluate your opinions about allergy in general, I urge you to consider speaking out about the need for a cure. Loud voices can really make a difference. It is important to consider the patient's point of view and not that of Big Pharma. These companies are important, but oftentimes they do not have your best interest at heart. That is not their job. Developing a cure would dry up their revenue streams like their medicines dry up our sinuses.

Americans spend upwards of 65 billion dollars every year just to treat their allergies. A cure would be life-changing for most of them. The disadvantaged segment of our population (many of whom suffer with symptoms because they can't afford to treat them) and those without access to insurance would benefit immensely, especially our children. A cure would eliminate the need for treatment. We need to convince important people, including our elected officials, that the words "My allergies are out of control" mean much more than simply, "Hand me another box of tissues."

Since I have no first-hand knowledge of procedures or progress in the field of scientific research, I am forced to be content with the few bits and pieces I can pull up on the internet. I can, however, express my wish list for the future. I wish someone would turn off the switch and teach our immune systems to change those monsters into friends. Even better, I wish for a vaccine which would block their appearance in the first place. To those who are working nonstop for a cure, I wish you Godspeed, and I wish the word "allergified" would become obsolete.

When I look back at how far I have come as an allergic individual, I liken my symptom-free status to that of a cure. My recent yearly physical resulted in a glowing report. All tests were in the normal range (bone density, EKG, cognitive, bloodwork, and so forth). My blood pressure was 120/80 and no medications were indicated. My dentist admires my cavity-free teeth and continues to be amazed by the results I achieve by flossing and brushing with coconut oil. I see Dr. Pienkowski regularly, twice a year. He checks me thoroughly and monitors my DHEA levels. I continue my injections every two weeks, and again, no medications are necessary. We achieved my cure the hard way, but we proved it can be done. I smile to myself as we both know what it means when I can still say with confidence, "I hardly ever sneeze."

Conclusion

#thisconclusionisjustanillusionitsabeginningnotanend

As this account of my allergic journey comes to a close, I look back with no regrets. You may wonder why I feel such a need to share this very personal story with strangers. Celebrating my success in silence would certainly have been much easier, but that is not who I am.

Allergy monsters robbed me of the ability to control the outcome of my best intentions. They robbed me of a successful career, regular church attendance, social activities, close friends, volunteer work, and important family events. Once these monsters met their match, my enthusiastic energy was restored, and now Michael and I enjoy traveling and entertaining. Our home is tidy, friends are welcome, and with the exception of an occasional chemical exposure, my emotions are steady and calm. Our beautiful story is based on a lifetime of faith, hope, determination, and love. It is a true testament to the fact that monsters can be slain, puzzles completed, mysteries solved, and mountains moved.

Emphasizing my long-awaited "normal" life is significant because now I can clearly demonstrate just how far we have come since that first long-ago conversation in Dr. Pienkowski's office. Every single aspect of my severe illness was indeed, allergy-related. This having been said, I need to make it clear that I am not advocating that everyone suffering from the "allergic achoos" arrive at an allergist's door, demanding that he or she "fix everything." That would be at the very least, unrealistic expectation. However, the prospect of a good prognosis is indeed very real.

Thinking back over the early years, I wish my Aunt Mary could still be here to finally understand why her precious darling girl woke up crying in the middle of the night. As she smiles down on us from Heaven, I hope you are smiling too, as you process my story, inspired by the facts. You, too, can achieve a non-allergified, symptom-free status, probably much more quickly than I did. My journey has been long, and extreme. By sharing my details in a compassionate manner, I hope I have spurred you on to find a qualified clinician who will treat your body as a whole entity, and customize a special treatment, just for you. As you begin your own journey, in search of an allergy-free, healthy, happy life, I wish you well. Don't let the monsters wear you down.

Now, about that marathon…

The End

Biography

Clyde Taliaferro Moore DeGraw, better known as Tollie, was born on June 6, 1947, in Cleveland, Tennessee. She studied at the University of North Carolina at Greensboro, The University of Tennessee, St. Nicholas Academy of London, and Memphis State University. She is the author of SECRET CITY, The Second Generation, and THE GUNNY, A Tribute to the Life of MGySgt. Jay W. DeGraw. She and her husband Michael have been happily married for over 50 years. Today they live a healthy life, free of medication, in Oak Ridge, Tennessee. Tollie is currently in the process of writing three more books.

www.ingramcontent.com/pod-product-compliance
Lightning Source LLC
Chambersburg PA
CBHW050805260726

48660CB00004B/1260